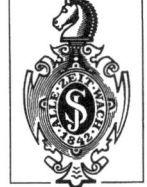

Jean-Noël Bruneton
and M. Benozio M. Bléry H. A. Gharbi
B. Senecail V. Tran-Minh

Ultrasonography of the Spleen

With Contributions by
C. Anagnostoupoulos C. Balu-Maestro M. Ben Cheikh
S. Chagnon P. Deffrenne J. Drouillard J.-G. Fuzibet
P. Jacquenod P. Marbot C.-H. Morin de Finfe
F. Normand J.-P. Pracros

With 100 Figures

Translated by N. Reed Rameau

Springer-Verlag
Berlin Heidelberg New York
London Paris Tokyo

Author

Dr. Jean-Noël Bruneton
Service de Radiologie, Centre Antoine-Lacassagne
36, Voie Romaine, 06054 Nice Cedex, France

Translator

Nancy Reed Rameau
Centre Antoine-Lacassagne
36, Voie Romaine, 06054 Nice Cedex, France

ISBN-13: 978-3-642-73201-0   e-ISBN-13: 978-3-642-73199-0
DOI: 10.1007/978-3-642-73199-0

Library of Congress Cataloging-in-Publication Data
Ultrasonography of the spleen / Jean-Noël Bruneton ... [et al.]; with contributions by
C. Anagnostoupoulos ... [et al.]; translated by N. Reed Rameau. p. cm. Includes
bibliographies and index.
ISBN-13: 978-3-642-73201-0 (Germany: est.)
1. Spleen-Diseases-Diagnosis. 2. Spleen-Imaging. 3. Diagnosis, Ultrasonic. I. Bruneton,
J. N. [DNLM: 1. Splenic Diseases-diagnosis. 2. Ultrasonic Diagnosis. WH 600 U47]
RC645.U445 1988 616.4'1-dc19 DNLM/DLC for Library of Congress 87-32195

© Springer-Verlag Berlin Heidelberg 1988
Softcover reprint of the hardcover 1st edition 1988

The use of registered names, trademarks, etc. in this publication does not imply, even in the
absence of a specific statement, that such names are exempt from the relevant protective
laws and regulations and therefore free for general use.

Product Liability: The publisher can give no guarantee for information about drug dosage
and application thereof contained in the book. In every individual case the respective user
must check its accuracy by consulting other pharmaceutical literature.

2121/3140-543210

Foreword

Only a few years ago, most treatises on sonography
covered all the diagnostic applications of ultrasound, de-
scribing organs from the brain down to the placenta. Dr.
Bruneton and his associates must be thanked for presenting this book devoted to the spleen. It probably offers
the most complete presentation of details and the richest
images available in its field. This book will thus become
the ultimate reference in most libraries of books on sonography.

March 1988   F. Weill

The authors wish to thank
Christine Rostagni, Françoise Fein, and Bernard Fontaine
for their assistance in the preparation of this book.

Contents

List of Contributors

Catherine Anagnostoupoulos
Service de Radiologie Centrale, Hôpital Lariboisière
2, Rue Ambroise Paré, 75010 Paris, France

Catherine Balu-Maestro
Service de Radiologie, Centre Antoine-Lacassagne
36, Voie Romaine, 06054 Nice Cedex, France

Mohamed Ben Cheikh
Service de Radiologie, Hôpital Militaire El Omrane
Tunis, Tunisia

Michel Benozio
Département d'Imagerie, Hôpital Charles Nicolle
1, Rue de Germont, 76031 Rouen Cedex, France

Michel Bléry
Service de Radiologie Centrale, Hôpital Lariboisière
2, Rue Ambroise Paré, 75010 Paris, France

Jean-Noël Bruneton
Service de Radiologie, Centre Antoine-Lacassagne
36, Voie Romaine, 06054 Nice Cedex, France

Sophie Chagnon
Service de Radiologie Centrale, Hôpital Lariboisière
2, Rue Ambroise Paré, 75010 Paris, France

Pierre Deffrenne
Service de Radiologie, Hôpital Debrousse
29, Rue Sœur-Bouvier, 69322 Lyon Cedex 02, France

Jacques Drouillard
Service de Radiologie, Hôpital du Haut-Lévêque
Avenue Magellan, 33600 Pessac, France

Jean-Gabriel Fuzibet
Service de Radiologie, Hôpital de Cimiez
4, Avenue Victoria, 06031 Nice, France

Hassen A. Gharbi
Service de Radiologie, Institut National de Santé de l'Enfance
Place Bab Saâdoun, 1007 Tunis Jabbari, Tunisia

Pascal Jacquenod
Service de Radiologie Centrale, Hôpital Lariboisière
2, Rue Ambroise Paré, 75010 Paris, France

Philippe Marbot
Service de Radiologie, Centre Hospitalier Territorial Gaston Bourret
Noumea, New Caledonia

Charles-Henri Morin de Finfe
Service de Radiologie, Hôpital Debrousse
29, Rue Sœur-Bouvier, 69332 Lyon Cedex 02, France

Frank Normand
Service de Radiologie, Centre Antoine-Lacassagne
36, Voie Romaine, 06054 Nice Cedex, France

Jean-Pierre Pracros
Service de Radiologie, Hôpital Debrousse
29, Rue Sœur-Bouvier, 69332 Lyon Cedex 02, France

Bernard Senecail
Unité d'Echo-scanographie viscérale, Hôpital Morvan
5, Avenue Foch, 29279 Brest Cedex, France

Van Tran-Minh
Service de Radiologie, Hôpital Debrousse
29, Rue Sœur-Bouvier, 69332 Lyon Cedex 02, France

1 Sonographic Anatomy of the Normal Spleen, Normal Anatomic Variants, and Pitfalls

B. SENECAIL

A lymphoreticular organ which arises as a mesenchymal bulge on the left side of the dorsal mesogastrium, the spleen is connected on a bypass basis to the portal system. In addition to its hematopoietic and hemolytic functions, this organ of the immune system is involved in combatting infections and removing toxins.

Many diseases affecting the spleen result in splenomegaly, the most frequent reason prompting exploration. The densely vascularized splenic pulp is particularly vulnerable to left upper quadrant trauma. Systemic examination of the spleen is thus advisable in all patients who have sustained blunt abdominal injury.

1.1 Anatomy of the Spleen

1.1.1 Morphology and Structure

The major treatises on splenic anatomy emphasize the variety of possible shapes: Testut and Jacob (1934) compared the spleen to a transversally flattened ovoid segment. Rouvière (1978) identified a polyhedric type, with four distinct surfaces, and an ovoid "coffee bean" type with only a convex surface and a flat surface, although the latter occasionally presents three facets, or flat surfaces. Based on a series of 100 dissections, Michels (1942) described three main configurations: an orange segment shape (44% of cases), a tetrahedral form (42%), and a triangular form (14%), which he divided into two major types: com-

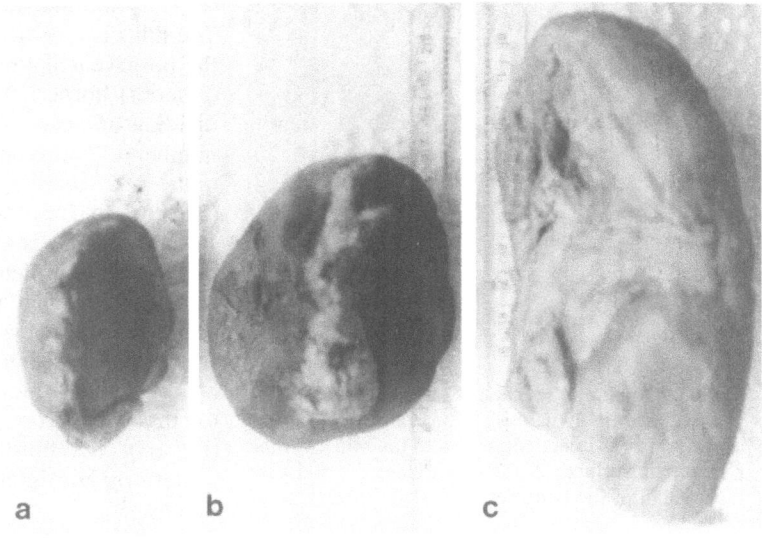

Fig. 1.1 a–c. Photographs of three normal spleens. **a** Small ovoid spleen. **b** Average-sized triangular spleen. **c** Large tetrahedral spleen

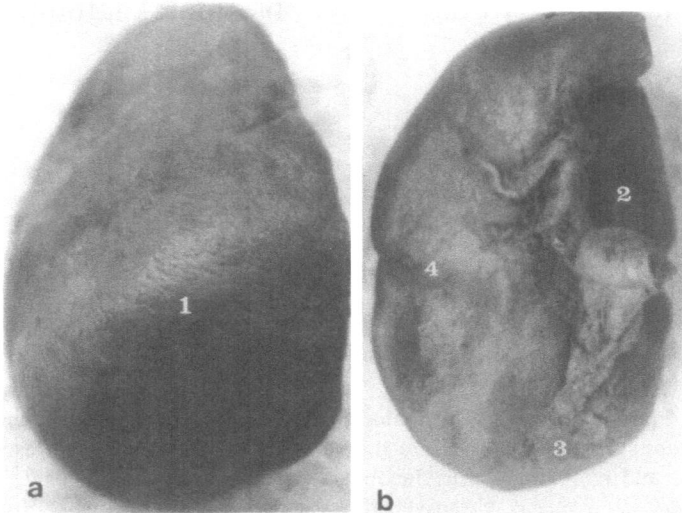

Fig. 1.2 a, b. External (**a**) and internal (**b**) views of a normal spleen showing the diaphragmatic *(1)*, gastric *(2)*, colic *(3)*, and renal *(4)* surfaces

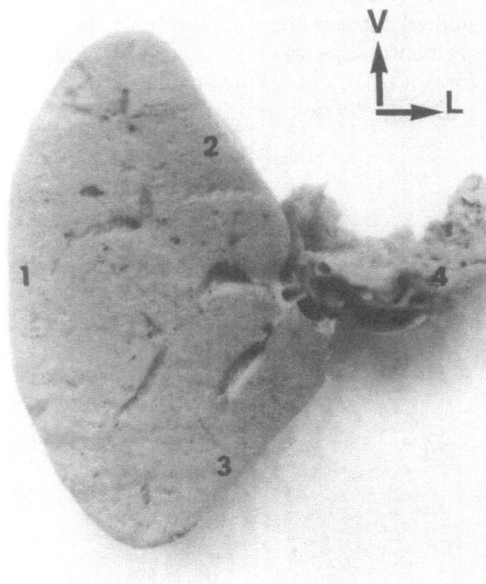

Fig. 1.3. Anatomic specimen: spleen dissected perpendicular to its long axis; the extremity of the tail of the pancreas is still connected to the hilus: *1*, diaphragmatic surface; *2*, gastric surface; *3*, renal surface; *4*, tail of the pancreas

pact spleens with a narrow hilus and even borders (30%) and "distributed" type spleens with a spread-out hilus (70%). Specimens photographed at the Laboratory of Anatomy in Brest, France (Figs. 1.1 and 1.2) illustrate this morphologic variability. However, it was always possible to identify at least two splenic surfaces: a convex, external surface and a concave (or flat) medial surface bearing the hilus. The hilus is a vertical fissure located closer to the posteromedial border than to the superior (anterior) border; the hilus is pierced by the dividing branches of the splenic artery, and a number of veins emerge from the hilus to unite at a variable distance from the spleen (2-6 cm) to form the splenic vein (Michels 1942). The hilus is also the site of insertion of the pancreaticosplenic omentum and the gastrosplenic ligament, peritoneal reflections continuous with the visceral peritoneum of the spleen. These features are well illustrated by an anatomic section prepared perpendicular to the long axis of a tetrahydral spleen (Fig. 1.3); the third, concave surface facing posteriorly and inferiorly is related to the left kidney.

While the gross anatomy of the splenic parenchyma is basically homogeneous, microscope examination reveals a complex histology: the

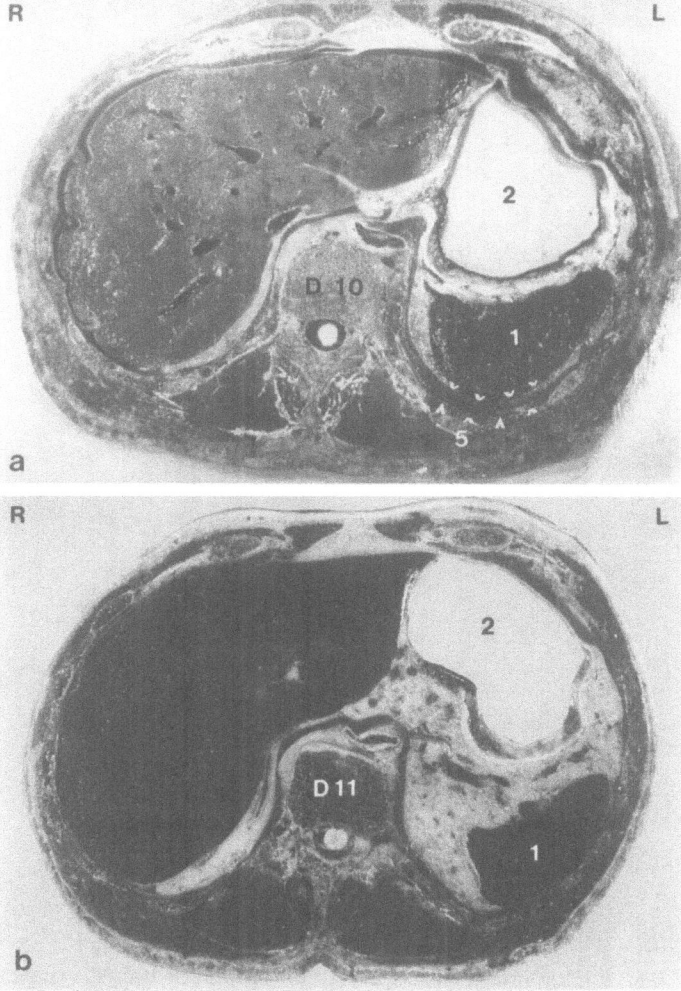

Fig. 1.4a, b. Photographs of two transverse abdominal sections at the level of D10 (**a**) and D11 (**b**), showing the morphology and the relations of the spleen: *1*, spleen; *2*, stomach; *3*, splenic pedicle extending over the tail of the pancreas; *4*, left retroperitoneal space; *5*, left pleural recess

spleen contains both white pulp (lymphoid areas surrounding the splenic arteries) and red pulp (a dense capillary network consisting of blood-filled pulp sinuses and pulp cords). Owing to its particular consistency, the spleen has been likened to a vascular "sponge," which explains its sensitivity to trauma.

Modern anatomic studies (Nguyen et al. 1982) have demonstrated the terminal and segmental nature of the intrasplenic arterial supply; these findings have served as the basis for controlled partial splenectomies and the conservative sur-

gical procedures advocated for children (Matsuyama et al. 1976).

1.1.2 Location and Relations of the Spleen

Situated in the left upper abdomen, the spleen lies deep within the left subphrenic bed, which is delimited by the contiguous organs. Serial transverse anatomic sections of the upper abdomen at the level of the tenth, eleventh, and twelfth dorsal vertebrae (Fig. 1.4) show the

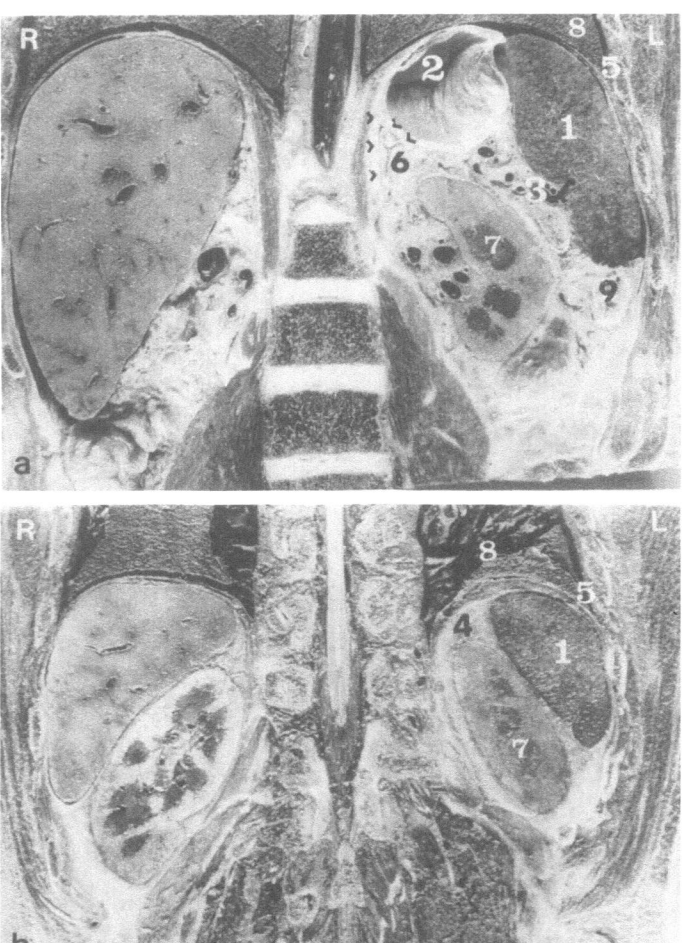

Fig. 1.5 a, b. Two frontal sections of the subphrenic beds showing the location of the spleen and the relations of its surfaces: *1 – 5*, as in Fig. 1.4; *6*, left suprarenal gland; *7*, left kidney; *8*, base of the left lung; *9*, left colic flexure

posterolateral or diaphragmatic surface of the spleen molding to the concave outline of the left hemidiaphragm.

Through the intermediary of this hemidiaphragm, the spleen is related to the base of the left lung; its cephalic border extends to the upper ninth rib; the caudal border lies at the level of the lower eleventh rib.

The *posteromedial surface* is related to the reretroperitoneal space containing the left adrenal gland and the left kidney, whose upper pole is the origin of this surface's concavity. A longitudinal section through the splenic bed reveals

that the organ is actually oriented backwards and downwards.

The *anterolateral or gastric surface* of the spleen is related, from top to bottom, to the greater curvature of the stomach, the body of the stomach (with the tail of the pancreas rising behind), and the left colic flexure (Fig. 1.5).

The relations of the spleen with the tail of the pancreas depend on the degree of development and the orientation of the caudal pancreas. For Michels (1942), the tail of the pancreas is in actual contact with the splenic hilus in 30% of individuals. The left prolongation of the lesser peritoneal cavity (omental bursa) lies anterior to the pancreas. The left colic flexure passes in front of a fourth splenic surface oriented anteroinferiorly, but this surface is not always clearly demarcated from the gastric surface.

The left phrenicocolic ligament ("sustentaculum lienis") serves as a supporting structure for the spleen. It may explain temporary retention of a splenic effusion in certain patients after blunt abdominal injury.

Completely protected behind the lower ribs, the normal spleen lies against the lateral thoracic wall. The long axis of this oval structure is in the line of the tenth rib, its true anatomic landmark. The spleen is oriented in an oblique direction, inferiorly, anteriorly, and laterally.

1.1.3 Average Dimensions of the Cadaver Spleen

Autopsy measurements include the length or height from the summit to the base, the maximum width at the base, and the thickness or distance between the surface of the examination table, with the spleen lying on its anterolateral (gastric) surface, and a parallel plane tangent to the external surface. Dimensions vary only slightly from one series to another: 13 cm, 8 cm, and 3-3.5 cm respectively for Testut and Jacob (1934) and 12 cm, 8 cm, and 4 cm for Rouvière (1978). These authors indicate a weight of 180-200 g for the exsanguine spleen, but this figure can only be considered an average in view of the considerable variation in weight (80-300 g) reported by Michels (1942).

In an attempt to obtain a more accurate picture, results for each of the two spleen types (compact and distributed) were compared for a series of 45 spleens examined at the Laboratory of Anatomy in Brest. Dimensions for the 28 distributed spleens were as follows: length 9.5-13 cm; width 4.5-8 cm; thickness 1.5-4.5 cm. Results for the 17 compact spleens were: length 5.5-8 cm; width 3.5-5.5 cm; thickness 2.5-5 cm.

Numerous factors affect splenic anatomy: for Testut and Jacob (1934), the spleen tends to be smaller in females than in males, and is subject to involution with aging. Radiologic-ana-

tomic studies (DeLand 1970; Rao and Wagner 1972) have corroborated the role of age and sex. Even digestion appears to influence the shape and size of the organ: when the stomach is full and the colon is empty, the spleen is shaped like an orange segment; by contrast, when the stomach is contracted and the colon is distended, the spleen takes on a tetrahedral shape (Michels 1942). In addition, a racial factor was identified by Moon (1928), who reported a higher proportion of small spleens in blacks than in whites.

1.1.4 Congenital Anomalies and Normal Variants

Aside from variants of the splenic pedicle, which are excluded from this text, the sonographer must be aware of several variations in splenic morphology and location. Absence of the spleen or, on the contrary, the presence of multiple splenules are also occasionally encountered.

1.1.4.1 Fissured Spleen

The deep fissure characteristic of such organs originates at the anterior border and continues over the two main surfaces (Fig. 1.6, p.6); this feature is actually just an exaggeration of one of the fissures normally present on the anterior border.

1.1.4.2 Lobulated Spleen (Gooding 1978)

The lobulated spleen presents several deep fissures which divide the organ into several lobes; the resultant appearance resembles that of the fetal kidney. Such lobulations can be considered a consequence of extreme fissuration.

1.1.4.3 Spleen with Two Hili

Frequent (60% of cases according to Michels 1942), such spleens have a second fissure for the passage of vascular elements; it may be located on any of the surfaces, including the diaphragmatic surface.

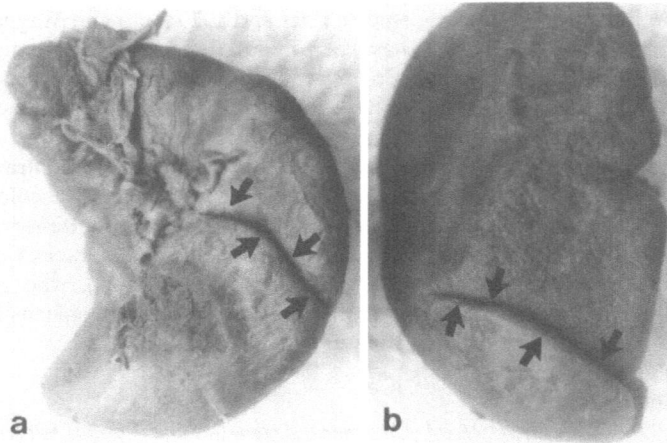

Fig. 1.6a, b. Two lobulated spleens: a deep fissure originating at the anterior border notches the medial surface (**a**) and the lateral surface (**b**)

1.1.4.4 Wandering or Ectopic Spleen (Hunter and Haber 1977; Lee et al. 1979; Michels 1942; Testut and Jacob 1934)

Normally, the spleen is held in place by the peritoneal reflections, the splenic pedicle, the phrenicocolic ligament and the adjacent viscera; organ mobility is thus limited to 3–4 cm. When the supporting structures become lax, as in very thin women or malnourished patients, the position of the spleen can vary considerably, depending on the subject's position. Moody and Van Nuys (1928), for example, reported splenic descent from the level of the upper half of the first lumbar vertebra to the fifth lumbar vertebra when patients changed from a lying down to a standing position. Wandering spleen has even been reported in the pelvis (Hatfield et al. 1976). Torsion of the elongated splenic pedicle is a possible complication, seen especially in women (Abell 1933; Salomonowitz et al. 1984).

1.1.4.5 Numeric Anomalies

While splenic agenesis, or congenital absence of the spleen, is very rare (Putschar and Manion 1956), multiple spleens are fairly common. Halpert and Eaton (1951), reporting on 600 autopsies, found 62 accessory spleens, an incidence slightly over 10%. The frequency in children was even higher (approximately 25%).

Accessory spleens tend to occur in the proximity of the main spleen, but they are also encountered on the pancreaticosplenic omentum, in the tail of the pancreas, in other peritoneal structures, and in the liver. They have even been reported in such distant sites as the scrotum (Bennett-Jones and St. Hill 1952). Of controversial origin, accessory spleens must not be confused with splenosis, a separate entity in which multiple implants of splenic tissue are dispersed throughout the peritoneal cavity, a possible consequence of splenic rupture (Curtis and Movitz 1946). The number of true supernumerary spleens varies from one to four elements. These small structures are usually no larger than a pea; the largest accessory spleen observed by Michels (1942) measured 2×3.5 cm. However, accessory spleens are subject to compensatory enlargement and can take over the functions of the normal spleen if the latter is injured or resected surgically (Pearson et al. 1978).

1.2 Ultrasonography of the Spleen

1.2.1 Equipment

Sector scanners with a small scan head are the ideal solution for splenic exploration as intercostal windows can be utilized. Linear transducers are generally unsuited for examination of the spleen except in patients with pronounced splenomegaly. Of course, real-time units offer the well-recognized advantages of rapidity and easy localization of the splenic pedicle. Manual scanners are particularly useful for measuring the long axis of certain enlarged spleens and for precise topographic evaluation of left upper quadrant masses because both intercostal and subcostal approaches are possible. Furthermore, their density resolution still remains slightly better than that of dynamic ultrasound equipment. The most commonly used frequencies for splenic examination are 3–3.5 MHz for adults and 4–5 MHz for children.

Focalization of the ultrasonic beam is helpful for detection of small intraparenchymal lesions, provided the transducer is adapted to the depth of the lesion: this necessitates a variable electronic focusing system or a battery of different transducers.

1.2.2 Patient Examination

As no preparation is required for ultrasonography, the technique can even be used in emergency situations. The only contraindications are subcutaneous gaseous emphysema and intolerance of contact with the transducer, encountered in certain trauma patients with rib fractures.

Patients can be examined in the supine position, but the right lateral decubitus position is preferable if the subject can be mobilized. The prone position is indicated only for exploration of very deep spleens, which are best explored by a lumbar approach. Examination of patients in a standing position allows assessment of splenic mobility and the organ's relations to adjacent viscera; the subdiaphragmatic nature of an effusion can also be determined in this manner, especially for patients incapable of deep inspiration. The left lateral decubitus position is indicated for investigation of small juxtasplenic collections, but is difficult to use for patients who have sustained left upper quadrant trauma. Evaluation of the relations of the spleen with the stomach, the tail of the pancreas, and the left adrenal gland

may be facilitated by having the patient drink fluid during the examination to distend the stomach.

1.2.3 Scanning Technique

The spleen can be scanned in several different ways:

- Intercostal scanning through the ninth, tenth, and eleventh left ribs allows semicircumferential exploration of the spleen.
- Recurrent views obtained by a left subcostal approach allow spleen construction along the anterior and anterolateral directions (the patient must be examined in deep inspiration).
- Anterior, lateral, and lumbar views obtained by combined intercostal/subcostal explorations.

Regardless of the examination approach, scans must first be obtained to construct the spleen along its long axis: this is generally done by orienting the beam parallel to the tenth rib, on both sides of the organ. Scans are then obtained perpendicular to the long axis, using the same acoustic window. The transducer is turned 90° and the beam is aimed upwards until the dome of the diaphragm is encountered; the beam is then angled downwards until the lower pole of the spleen is passed.

Certain examiners (Holm et al. 1976; Taboury 1980) perform sonography without regard to splenic orientation, using strictly sagittal and transverse scans of the left upper quadrant. Data obtained in this manner may be easier to interpret, but such scans may fail to evaluate the organ's true maximum dimensions.

1.3 Sonographic Features of the Normal Spleen

1.3.1 Splenic Contour

The contour of the spleen is sharply defined as a simple interface along the visceral surfaces and as a high amplitude interface at points of contact with the dome of the diaphragm. Construction of the superior (posterior) contour may be defective if the patient does not

breathe deeply enough; the same problem occurs with certain types of transducers when
aerated pulmonary parenchyma is interposed
between the probe and the top of the dome
(Weill 1980).

The spleen normally has a smooth contour, except for the characteristic serrated or draped
appearance of the anterior border.

A double splenic contour reflects the pathologic interposition of fluid between the outer
limit of the splenic parenchyma and the mal-
pighian capsule, or between this capsule and
the visceral peritoneum that is normally continuous with it.

1.3.2 Echo Pattern of the Splenic Parenchyma

Apart from possible intraparenchymal prolon-
gations of the hilus and vascular elements, the
spleen has a homogeneous echo structure: its
moderate echo density is higher than that of
the renal parenchyma, slightly lower than or
the same as that of the liver, and markedly
lower than that of the pancreas. Whereas
with first generation ultrasound instruments
(2 MHz) the normal splenic tissue appeared to
have a very low echodensity, or was even considered sonolucent (Weill 1980), the improved
axial, lateral, and densitometric resolution of
state-of-the-art equipment today reveals this
organ to be mildly echogenic. Response to
variation of the gain is similar to that for hepatic tissue: the echogenicity rises gradually as
the gain is increased and can even reach satu-
ration.

1.3.3 Analysis of Splenic Sonograms

1.3.3.1 Scans Parallel to the Long Axis

Such scans visualize the spleen as a semioval,
crescent-shaped, or elongated droplet structure: the convex superior border corresponds
to the diaphragmatic surface while the slightly
concave inferior border represents the gastro-
colic surface. The maximum cephalocaudal
dimension measured on these scans corresponds to the length described in anatomic
treatises, provided that measurement is made
from the most cephalad point of the diaphrag-

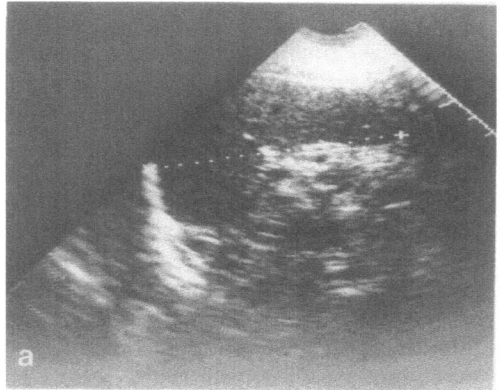

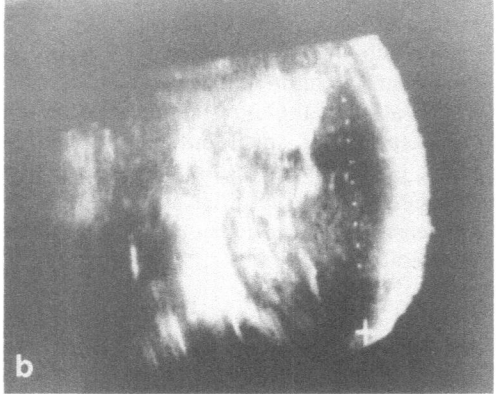

Fig. 1.7 a, b. Sonographic appearance of the normal
spleen: scan parallel to the long axis (**a**) and scan
perpendicular to the long axis (**b**)

matic surface to the inferior border of the
spleen (Fig. 1.7 a).

1.3.3.2 Scans Perpendicular to the Long Axis

The spleen is imaged as a triangular structure,
analogous to the corresponding anatomic section: the convex lateral border corresponds to
the diaphragmatic surface, the slightly concave
anteromedial border represents the gastric surface, and the concave posteromedial border is
related to the left kidney (Fig. 1.7 b). The anteroposterior dimension on these scans differs
somewhat from the width mentioned in anatomic studies, because sonographic evaluation
of the distance between the superior border
and the posteromedial border only gives the
width of the gastric surface. Similarly, ultra-

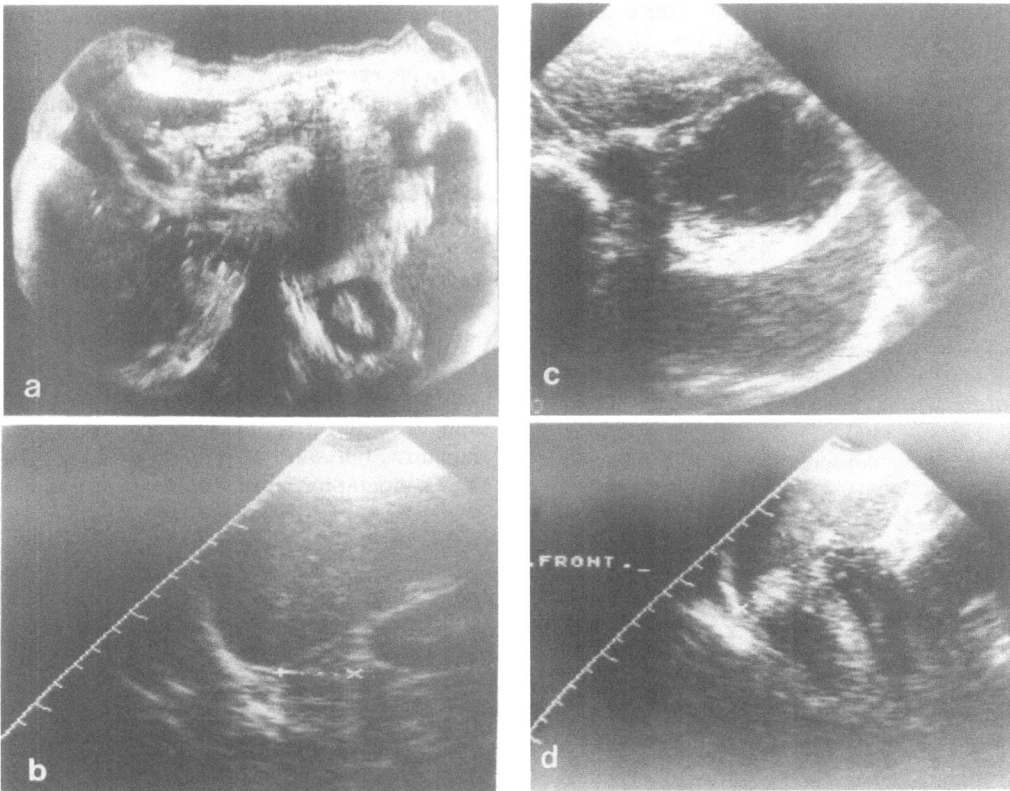

Fig. 1.8 a–d. Sonographic appearance of splenic relations: **a** with the left kidney; **b** with the left suprarenal gland; **c** with the stomach; **d** with the tail of the pancreas

sonic determination of the distance from the superior to the posterolateral border will include a certain degree of error if the beam has not been oriented in a strictly orthogonal manner. Nevertheless, organ thickness determined from sonograms will closely approximate anatomic reality provided that the scans used clearly demonstrate all three surfaces. Width thus cannot be measured on scans taken too cephalad, as the spleen will appear crescent-shaped rather than triangular (Fig. 1.8).

1.3.4 Sonographic Splenometry

Although several authors have defined normal values for the adult spleen, neither the methodology nor the type of measurements are standardized (Holm et al. 1976; Koga and Morikawa 1975; Taboury 1980; Weill 1980).

The upper limits of normal thus vary from 12–14 cm for the long axis, 6–12 cm for the width, and 4–8 cm for the thickness.

In a prospective study conducted over a twelve-month period, 170 healthy adults of both sexes were examined using the procedure described in Section 1.3.3. The study population was divided into two groups as a function of age (younger or older than 50 years). Table 1.1 lists both the average calculated values and the maximum values actually measured for each of the three dimensions. The small difference between the average and maximum lengths is probably due to the high proportion of distributed spleens in the study population. Study findings confirmed the small values reported for the transverse dimension. As shown by Table 1.1, this data obtained in living individuals concurs well with autopsy measurements.

10   B. Senecail

Table 1.1. Dimensions (in cm) of the normal adult spleen in a group of 170 individuals

	18 to 50 years		Over 50 years	
	M	F	M	F
Cephalocaudal dimension				
Calculated average	11.82	10.97	9.75	9.10
Maximum measured	13.00	12.60	10.70	10.50
Anteroposterior dimension				
Calculated average	6.86	6.10	6.01	6.12
Maximum measured	8.50	7.50	7.00	6.60
Transverse dimension				
Calculated average	3.84	3.80	3.46	2.98
Maximum measured	5.10	5.20	4.10	3.50

Table 1.2. Dimensions of the long axis of the spleen in a series of 50 children

At birth:	35 ± 2 mm
Between 2 and 3 years:	65 ± 5 mm
Between 4 and 7 years:	80 ± 8 mm
Between 8 and 13 years:	90 ± 10 mm
Between 14 and 17 years:	105 ± 13 mm

Owing to the lack of references concerning variations in splenic size during childhood, the long axis of the spleen was systematically measured by ultrasound in a group of 50 children free of any splenic pathology with harmonious pondostatural development normal for their age. The small population precludes establishment of size charts, but Table 1.2 provides useful indication of size variations in children. The dispersion of values increases with the appearance of sexual dimorphism, and individual factors of variation become apparent especially after the third stage of childhood.

1.3.5 Sonographic Pitfalls

1.3.5.1 Splenic Ectopia

Mentioned as a "curiosity" by Weill (1980), a spleen lying anterior to the kidney can mimic a prerenal pseudotumor. Failure to correctly identify such a structure usually means that the patient will undergo computed tomographic examination at the very least, if not more aggressive procedures.

Sonographic diagnosis of an ectopic spleen is based on visualization of a structure with the sonographic and morphologic features of the spleen and demonstration of an empty left subphrenic bed, without its normal parenchymal contents. When doubt persists, a multiposition ultrasound examination, including Trendelenburg's position where appropriate, should permit accurate diagnosis.

The presence of both a normal spleen and an ectopic accessory spleen can prove more difficult to identify; sonography can suggest the diagnosis but will not provide positive proof. The sonographer must also keep in mind the fact that the spleen may be located on the right side in individuals with situs inversus (cf. Chapter 2).

1.3.5.2 The Lobulated Spleen

Exploration of spleens with a deep fissure involves two diagnostic problems: the image may be confused with a laceration in patients who have sustained blunt abdominal trauma (Moss et al. 1983) or be mistaken for a juxtasplenic mass of gastric or suprarenal origin (Kuhns and Seeger 1983). Care must also be taken not to mistake the normal serrated appearance of the superior splenic border for pathologic nodules: absence of an altered tissue echo pattern opposite these nodular images is a basic feature ruling out a pathologic process.

1.3.5.3 Accessory Spleens

While accessory spleens are relatively frequent, they involve few diagnostic problems. In fact, their small size often precludes sonographic detection (Holm et al. 1976). The only problem for differential diagnosis occurs with accessory spleens attaining 2-3 cm (Fig. 1.9).

Adenopathies of the splenic pedicle (Fig. 1.10) are the major differential diagnosis, as these structures have the same location, nodular form and small dimensions as accessory spleens. Diagnosis can be especially difficult if the clinical context is noncontributory, in particular because the relatively low echogenicity of lymph nodes does not allow differentiation from a splenic structure. In such cases, identification of an accessory spleen may require comparison of the spontaneous density and the postcontrast density of the structure with

that of the normal splenic parenchyma (Bagni et al. 1983; Fig. 1.11).

An accessory spleen may be misdiagnosed as a nodular mass arising from the suprarenal gland or the upper pole of the left kidney; the opposite error is also possible (Kuhns and Seeger 1983; Moss et al. 1983). Tumors of the

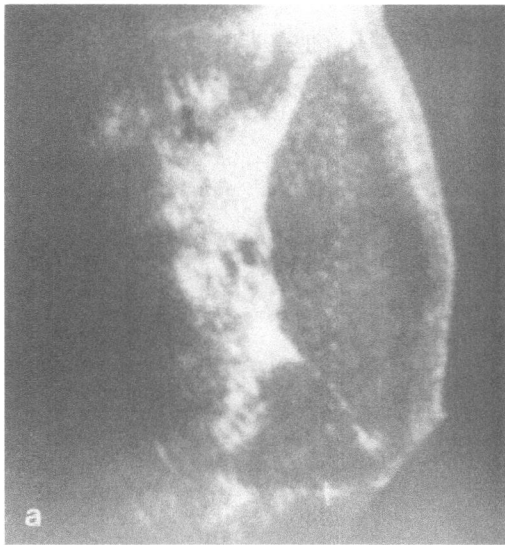

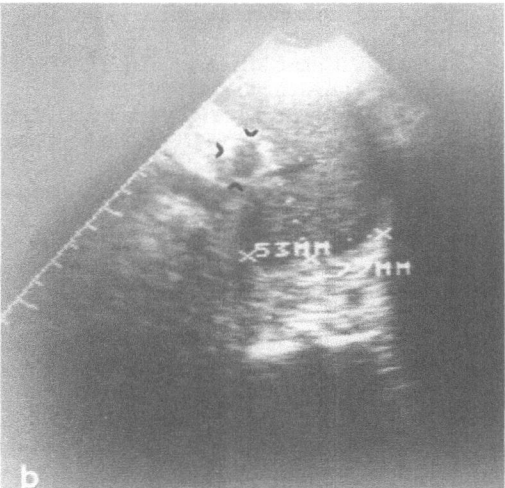

Fig. 1.9 a, b. Sonographic appearance of a lobulated spleen

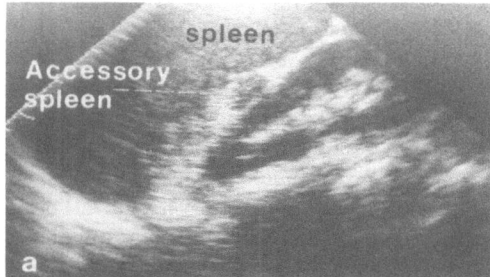

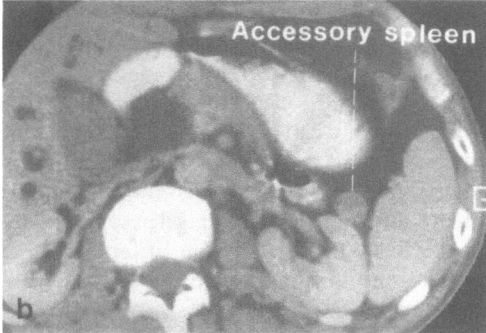

Fig. 1.10 a, b. Sonographic (a) and computed tomographic (b) appearance of the same accessory spleen, lying anterior to the left kidney and in contact with the normal spleen

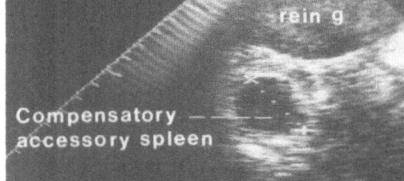

Fig. 1.11. Small compensatory spleen that developed from an accessory spleen in a patient splenectomized 5 years earlier. *rein g,* left kidney

tail of the pancreas involve fewer diagnostic problems as they are usually larger than accessory spleens. After splenectomy, an accessory spleen may enlarge as the result of a compensatory phenomenon (Beahrs and Stephens 1980; Pearson et al. 1978).

1.4 Conclusion

1.4.1 Quantitative Sonographic Criteria

Like Weill (1980), we feel that at least two dimensions must be taken into account before speaking of splenomegaly: this prevents errors created by distributed spleens which have a fairly long axis but are not very thick. Possible splenomegaly is probably best evaluated by considering the cephalocaudal and the maximum transverse diameters. The anteroposterior diameter tends to vary in the same manner as the cephalocaudal dimension, and sonographic evaluation often includes a degree of error.

Splenomegaly can be considered present when the spleen measures over 13 cm in long axis *and* 5 cm or more in transverse diameter in males under 50 years of age. These limits drop respectively to 12 and 5 cm in females under age 50, and to 11 and 4 cm in both sexes after 50 years of age.

1.4.2 Qualitative Sonographic Criteria

Regardless of the sections obtained, splenic sonograms should always include at least one concave - or flat - surface. Any significant convexity involving an entire visceral surface (gastric, colic, or renal) is indicative of pathologic deformation.

The borders of the normal spleen are always sharply defined, never double. The splenic tissue must have a homogeneous echo pattern, and be slightly less echogenic than the normal liver. Homogeneity must be conserved even at high gain settings.

A small swelling or even a deep notch are not pathologic provided they occur on the anterior border *and* there is no concomitant alteration in the echo pattern or echo density of the adjacent parenchyma.

There are no formal diagnostic criteria for accessory spleens, but these generally small (less than 4 cm) structures have an echo pattern identical to that of the regular spleen and tend to occur near this organ, from the hilus to the tail of the pancreas.

1.5 References

Abell I (1933) Wandering spleen with torsion of the pedicle. Ann Surg 98: 722-735

Bagni P, Belloir A, Rhomer P, Weill F (1983) Les rates accessoires. Etude scanographique et ultrasonore. J Radiol 64: 43-46

Beahrs JR, Stephens DH (1980) Enlarged accessory spleens: CT appearance in postsplenectomy patients. AJR 135: 483-486

Bennett-Jones MJ, St Hill CA (1952) Accessory spleen in the scrotum. Br J Surg 40: 259-262

Curtis GM, Movitz D (1946) The surgical significance of the accessory spleen. Ann Surg 123: 276-298

DeLand FH (1970) Normal spleen size. Radiology 97: 589-592

Gooding GAW (1978) The ultrasonic and computed tomographic appearance of splenic lobulations: a consideration in the ultrasonic differential of masses adjacent to the left kidney. Radiology 126: 719-720

Halpert B, Eaton WL (1951) Accessory spleens: a pilot study of 600 necropsies. Anat Rec 4: 109-111

Hatfield PM, Clouse ME, Cady B (1976) Ectopic pelvic spleen. Arch Surg 111: 603-605

Holm HH, Kristenssen JK, Rasmussen SN, Pedersen JF, Hancke S (eds) (1976) Abdominal ultrasound. Munksgaard, Copenhagen

Hunter TB, Haber K (1977) Sonographic diagnosis of a wandering spleen. AJR 129: 925-926

Koga T, Morikawa Y (1975) Ultrasonographic determination of the splenic size and its clinical usefulness in various liver diseases. Radiology 115: 157-161

Kuhns LR, Seeger J (eds) (1983) Atlas of computed tomography variants. Year Book Medical Publishers, Chicago

Lee TG, Brickman FE, Satterwhite GR, Avecilla LS (1979) Ultrasound demonstration of wandering spleen. Arch Surg 114: 13-15

Matsuyama S, Suzuki N, Nagamachi Y (1976) Rupture of the spleen in the newborn: treatment without splenectomy. J Pediatr Surg 11: 115-116

Michels NA (1942) The variational anatomy of the spleen and splenic artery. Am J Anat 70: 21-72

Moody RO, Van Nuys RG (1928) Some results of a study of roentgenograms of the abdominal viscera. AJR 20: 348-353

Moon VH (1928) Racial variations in size of spleen. Arch Pathol 5: 1040–1046

Moss AA, Gamsu G, Genant HK (eds) (1983) Computed tomography of the body. Saunders, Philadelphia

Nguyen Huu N, Person H, Hong R, Valée B, Nguyen Hoan V (1982) Anatomical approach to the vascular segmentation of the spleen (lien) based on controlled experimental partial splenectomies. Anat Clin 4: 265–277

Pearson HA, Johnston D, Smith KA, Touloukian RJ (1978) The born-again spleen: return of splenic function after splenectomy for trauma. N Engl J Med 298: 1389–1392

Putschar WGJ, Manion WC (1956) Congenital absence of the spleen and associated anomalies. Am J Clin Pathol 26: 429–470

Rao UVG, Wagner HN Jr (1972) Normal weights of human organs. Radiology 102: 337–339

Rouvière H (1978) Anatomie humaine. Descriptive, topographique et fonctionnelle. Vol 2. 11th edn. Masson, Paris, pp 469–474

Salomonowitz E, Frick MP, Lund G (1984) Radiologic diagnosis of wandering spleen complicated by splenic volvulus and infarction. Gastrointest Radiol 9: 57–59

Taboury J (1980) Guide pratique d'échographie abdominale. Masson, Paris, pp 77–83

Testut L, Jacob O (1934) Traité d'anatomie topographique avec applications médico-chirurgicales. Vol 2. 5th edn. Douin, Paris, pp 123–141

Weill F (1980) L'ultrasonographie en pathologie digestive. Vigot, Paris, pp 459–471

2 Congenital Anomalies of the Spleen

V. Tran-Minh, J. P. Pracros, P. Deffrenne, C. H. Morin de Finfe

Congenital anomalies of the spleen can be divided into seven major categories:

1. Situs inversus (dextrosplenia)
2. Asplenia
3. Polysplenia
4. Wandering spleen
5. Splenogonadal fusion
6. Accessory spleen
7. Splenoma

Only the first five categories are dealt with in this chapter. Accessory spleens are usually considered normal variants (cf. Chapter 1), even though 10% of cases are associated with other congenital anomalies and there are several specific pathologic complications (trauma, acute torsion, infarction, compensatory hypertrophy after splenectomy). Likewise, splenomas (hamartomas) are often regarded as a particular type of benign tumor (cf. Chapter 4).

2.1 Situs Inversus

Situs inversus viscerum, or visceral heterotaxia, can occur either alone or in combination with other malformations (Hines and Eggum 1961; Tonkin and Tonkin 1982).

2.1.1 Uncomplicated Situs Inversus

2.1.1.1 Total Situs Inversus

Total situs inversus refers to mirror image positioning of the organs and vessels. The heart is to the right of the midline (dextrocardia); the positions of all of its chambers are reversed. The aorta turns to the right. There are three pulmonary lobes on the right and two on the left. The thoracic duct and the stomach are on the right; the gallbladder and the liver are on the left. The hepatic flexure is on the left; the splenic flexure is on the right. The cecum is in the left iliac fossa. All of the asymmetric vessels (such as the vena cavae) are reversed. The spleen is normal, but lies on the right. The splenic hilus faces to the left, with its superolateral aspect lying against the structure serving as the right kidney.

A rare entity (1 in 10000–20000 autopsies), total situs inversus is often latent, and not detected until adulthood. Many affected individuals are unaware of their condition, although two signs are suggestive:

- A right testicle lower than the left, a very common feature
- A counterclockwise hair whorl

Total situs inversus can be an incidental finding on sonograms, when an oval parenchymal mass demonstrated in the right upper quadrant presents all of the usual characteristics of a spleen: large superomedial pole, tapered inferolateral extremity, medial hilus, arterial and venous pedicle.

2.1.1.2 Partial Situs Inversus

Individuals with partial situs inversus present a combination of normal and reversed asymmetries: inversion may be limited to the thorax, to the cardiac chamber, or to transposition of the stomach. To our knowledge, there have been no reports of solitary splenic inversion.

2.1.2 Complicated Situs Inversus

Total situs inversus may be complicated by other malformation syndromes such as Kartagener's triad (a familial condition associating total situs inversus, abnormal paranasal sinuses, and bronchiectasis), asplenia, polysplenia, or isolated cardiac defects. The prognosis depends on the severity of anomalies.

Table 2.1. Main features of asplenia and polysplenia

Characteristic	Asplenia	Polysplenia
Relative frequency	+ + +	=
Sex	M > > F	M = F
Cardiac failure	+ + +	+ / −
Mortality before 1 year	+ + + +	+ +
Defect		
Bilateral superior venae cavae	+ + +	+ +
Interruption of inferior vena cava with azygos continuation	0	+ + +
Absent coronary sinus	+	+
Total anomalous pulmonary venous drainage	+ + + +	0
Right atrial and left atrial venous return separate	0	+ + +
Transposition of great vessels	+ + +	+
Pulmonary artery atresia or stenosis	+ + +	+
Dextrocardia	+	+
Single atrium	+ + +	+ + +
Single ventricle	+ + + +	+ + +
Trilobed lungs	+ + +	0
Bilobed lungs	0	+ + +
Eparterial bronchi	+ + +	0
Hyparterial bronchi	0	+ + +
Increased pulmonary vasculature	0	+ + +
Abdominal heterotaxia	+ + +	+ +
Horizontal liver	+ + +	+
Intestinal malrotation	+	+ +
Discordance between cardiac apex and gastric air bubble	+ +	+
Inferior vena cava and descending aorta on same side of spine	+ +	+
Absent gallbladder and/or biliary duct atresia	0	+
Urinary malformations	+	+
Horseshoe adrenal glands	+	0
Howell-Jolly bodies	+ + +	0

2.2 Asplenia (Table 2.1)

Asplenia, or congenital absence of the spleen, can be divided into two categories. Simple *agenesis of the spleen,* with or without malformations sparing the heart and body symmetry, accounts for around 25% of cases. The most characteristic anomaly associated with simple asplenia is microgastria: a tubular stomach without a distinct fundus located on the midline (Kessler and Smulewicz 1973). *Asplenia syndrome,* which represents the other 75% of cases, combines asplenia with defects in body symmetry and cardiac malformations (Putschar and Manion 1956a). Approximately 200 cases of this syndrome were reported in 1972 (Van Mierop et al. 1972). Male predominance is marked (two-thirds of cases). Neonatal cardiac failure is a major presenting symptom, and the mortality rate in the first year of life exceeds 95%. Asplenia syndrome has even been encountered in children with a rudimentary spleen.

Possible accompanying anomalies are described hereunder.

2.2.1 Bronchopulmonary Abnormalities

Right thoracic isomerism occurs in nearly 100% of cases. The right and left lungs each have three lobes (bilateral trilobed lungs). The left and right bronchus are located above the corresponding pulmonary artery (bilateral eparterial bronchi; Fig. 2.1). Plain chest radiographs will demonstrate:

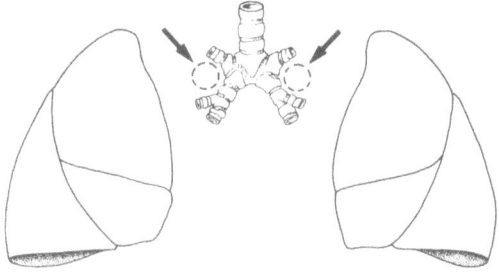

Fig. 2.1. Asplenia and right isomerism. Each lung has three lobes, like a normal right lung. The bronchi are eparterial, in other words they pass over the corresponding pulmonary artery *(arrow).* (After Van Mierop et al. 1972)

- A minor fissure on both the right and left lungs
- Right and left mainstem bronchi of comparable length
- Nonvisualization of the pulmonary arteries on lateral radiographs owing to their position posterior to the tracheobronchial tree (Soto et al. 1978)

2.2.2 Liver

Isomerism of the liver occurs in 50%–60% of cases. The liver has two symmetrical lobes and lies horizontally across both upper quadrants. The condition is readily identified by both sonography and CT (Freedom and Fellows 1973; Freedom and Treves 1973; Rao et al. 1982). Arteriograms may demonstrate absence of the celiac trunk and its branches. Arterial opacification of the liver takes place through a hepatic artery arising from the superior mesenteric artery; it probably corresponds to an arc of Buhler that has remained permeable. Exceptionally, the liver may be ectopic, lying in a site such as the adrenal gland (Rose et al. 1975).

2.2.3 Gallbladder

The gallbladder is usually located on the right; it rarely lies on the midline, even when the liver is on the midline. Agenesis of the gallbladder is also possible.

2.2.4 Stomach, Pancreas, Duodenum

The stomach is to the right of the midline in slightly over 50% of cases; exceptionally it lies on the midline or in the lower posterior mediastinum (Gray and Skandalakis 1972). The first and second parts of the duodenum, like the pancreas, often follow the movements of the stomach. A case of an annular pancreas has been reported.

2.2.5 Intestinal Anomalies

Malrotation of gut is common, with a vertical mesentery and only slight retroperitonealiza-tion. The colon may be completely free and lie inferior and posterior to the small intestine. Imperforate anus is a rare possibility.

2.2.6 Genitourinary Anomalies

Urinary malformations (horseshoe kidney, double collecting system, cystic kidney) are not common, but can easily be demonstrated by sonography.

2.2.7 Endocrine Glands

Malformations of the endocrine glands are rare, but rather characteristic, in particular fused "horseshoe" adrenal glands and agenesis of the left adrenal gland (Freedom 1972).

2.2.8 Musculoskeletal Anomalies

The incidence of skeletal and central nervous system anomalies is comparable to that of the general population, although the frequency of scoliosis is minimally elevated.

2.2.9 Biologic Anomalies

Peripheral blood smears will demonstrate Howell-Jolly bodies in red blood cells, reflecting the absence of functional splenic tissue.

2.2.10 Cardiovascular Anomalies

Cardiovascular anomalies are by far the most frequent and most severe accompanying malformations (Fig. 2.2). The association of asplenia – congenital cardiac disease – partial situs inversus is referred to as Ivemark's syndrome.

2.2.10.1 Systemic Veins

Two-thirds of patients have bilateral superior venae cavae (one on the right, one on the left); the remaining third have a single superior vena cava, either on the right or on the left. Van Mierop et al. (1972) reported six cases in

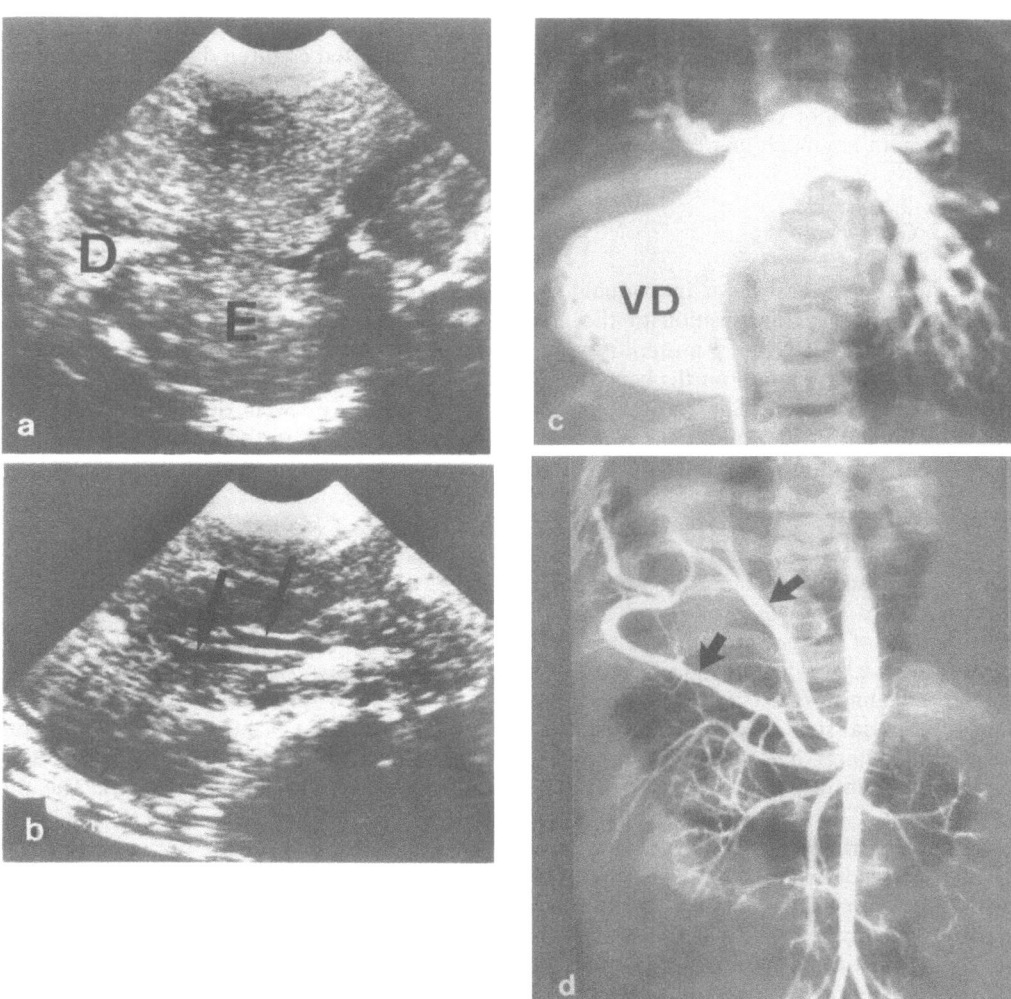

Fig. 2.2a-d. Asplenia in a 4-month-old infant with complex cardiovascular malformations and right pulmonary sequestration due to diaphragmatic eventration. **a** Recurrent right subcostal scan. The liver is bilobed, and a segment protrudes through an eventration *(E); D,* diaphragm. **b** Oblique right subcostal scan: presence of two abnormal vascular pedicles *(arrows)* coursing toward the eventration.

c Angiocardiography. The heart is on the *right,* with dextroversion. No visible inferior right pulmonary artery; *VD,* right ventricle. **d** Abdominal aortography. No splenic artery or splenic tissue visible. Presence of two abnormal systemic arteries *(arrows)* arising from the right side of the subphrenic aorta and coursing toward the sequestration

which the inferior vena cava was accompanied, on the contralateral side, by a common hepatic vein draining the corresponding lobe of the liver. This arrangement reflects bilateral persistence of the most proximal embryonic vitelline veins. This common hepatic vein is sometimes visible on angiograms; it can be demonstrated sonographically in patients with congenital interruption of the inferior vena cava. Azygos continuation of the inferior vena cava is rare. Location of the abdominal aorta and the inferior vena cava on the same side of the spine (either on the right or on the left) is a characteristic feature (Elliott et al. 1966; Tonkin and Tonkin 1982).

2.2.10.2 Pulmonary Veins

Total anomalous pulmonary venous return occurs in over 80% of cases. Partial and mixed venous return are much less common.

2.2.10.3 Great Vessels

Approximately two-thirds of individuals with asplenia also have transposition of the great vessels (anterior aorta and posterior pulmonary trunk). Nearly three-fourths have pulmonary atresia or stenosis. The aortic arch is located on the left in 70% of cases.

2.2.10.4 Heart

The cardiac apex is located on the right in over one-third of cases. Both atria have the morphology of a right atrium, and the coronary sinus is absent: such right isomerism of the atria is almost constant. Large defects occur in the atrial septum (septum primum and secondum defects in two-thirds of patients, septum primum defects only in one-third). In extreme cases there is only a single atrium ("common" atrium). The exact position of the atrium can be determined by scintigraphy (Fitzer 1976). Over 85% of patients have a common atrioventricular valve. Complete persistence of the atrioventricular canal with cor biloculare occurs in almost all cases. There is only one functioning ventricle, and it usually has the morphology of a right ventricle. Presence of a single coronary artery has also been reported.

2.3 Polysplenia (Table 2.1)

Polysplenia, an anomaly characterized by a multilobate spleen, is often associated in situs inversus with left isomerism and congenital heart defects. Polysplenia must be distinguished from accessory spleens and from the nodules of splenosis that can occur after trauma and subsequent splenectomy. The polysplenia syndrome is probably two to three times less common than asplenia; both sexes are affected similarly. Although the prognosis

is better than for asplenia (Rose et al. 1975), 60% of affected children die in the first year of life.

2.3.1 Gross Anatomy

The spleen may present marked lobulation. The organ usually consists of two distinct main lobules measuring 1–3 cm in diameter plus a number of smaller masses. Occasionally, there are 2–15 splenules of comparable size. Sonography will demonstrate polysplenia as a cluster of well delimited, hypoechoic rounded nodules in the upper right quadrant, usually along the greater curvature of the stomach. On rare occasions, the autonomous vascular pedicles of these nodules can be visualized during real-time examination.

2.3.2 Associated Noncardiovascular Malformations

Sixty-five percent of affected individuals present left pulmonary isomerism (bilobed lungs and hypoarterial bronchi; Fig. 2.3). The pulmonary vasculature is increased (Randall et al. 1973). The location of the liver varies: on the midline (26% of cases), on the right (31%), or on the left (43%). The gallbladder lies on the left just as often as on the right; midline locations are rarer. Contrary to popular belief, agenesis of the gallbladder is not pathognom-

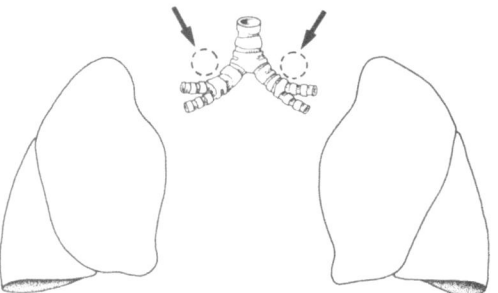

Fig. 2.3. Polysplenia and left isomerism. Each lung has two lobes, like a normal left lung. The bronchi are hyperarterial, in other words they pass under the corresponding pulmonary artery *(arrows)*. (After Van Mierop et al. 1972)

onic for polysplenia: it occurs in the asplenia syndrome and in healthy normal subjects as well. However, atresia of the bile ducts may occur with or without agenesis of the gallbladder (Chandra 1974).

The stomach is generally on the right (66% of cases), and determines the position of the pancreas and the first and second parts of the duodenum. Malrotation of gut is common (80% of cases).

The digestive tract arteries include a common celiomesenteric trunk with persistence of the ventral longitudinal anastomosis (arc of Buhler type). The origin of the splenic arteries is variable: one or more arteries may arise from the common trunk, the right gastroepiploic artery, or directly from the right side of the aorta (Curet et al. 1980; Vaughan et al. 1971).

No significant association has been reported between polysplenia and urogenital, musculoskeletal, or CNS malformations. There are no Howell-Jolly bodies in peripheral blood smears (Khattar et al. 1972).

2.3.3 Associated Cardiovascular Anomalies
(Figs. 2.4 and 2.5)

2.3.3.1 Venae Cavae

When there is a single vena cava, it tends to lie on the right more often than on the left. Bilateral venae cavae are frequent in individuals with polysplenia (43%). Congenital absence of the hepatic segment of the inferior vena cava is even more characteristic (70% of cases); drainage occurs by a right or left azygos continuation. Plain anteroposterior chest radiographs will demonstrate:

- A pseudotumoral left paravertebral mass
- A prominent azygos vein mimicking an aortic knob
- Occasionally, deviation of the left paravertebral line and dilatation of the left superior intercostal vein

Lateral radiographs obtained with the patient in deep inspiration will reveal absence of the posterior edge of the terminal inferior vena cava (Floyd and Nelson 1976; Haswell and Berrigan 1976; Heller et al. 1971; Vaughan et al. 1971).

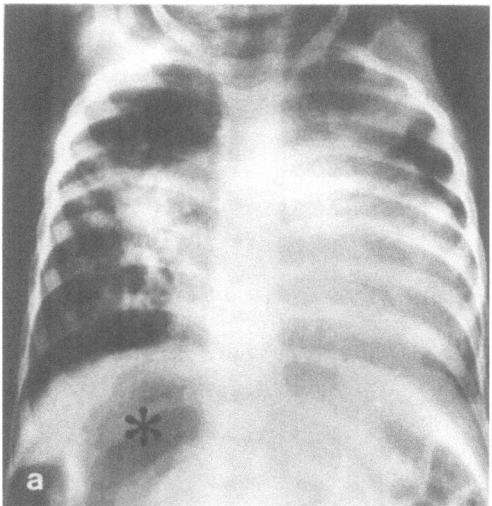

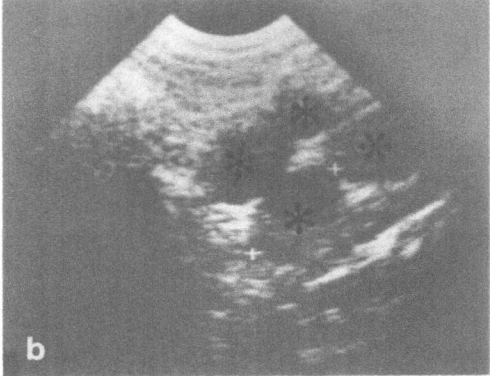

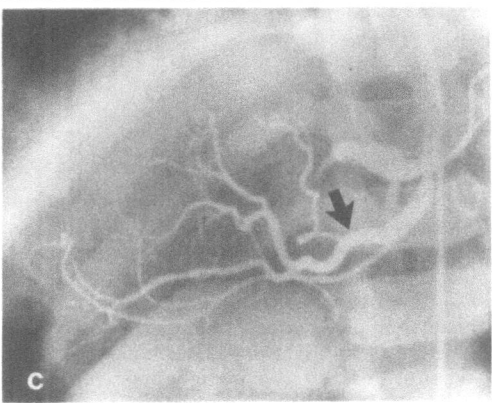

Fig. 2.4a-c. Polysplenia in a 2-year-old child with a complex cardiopathy and visceral situs inversus (patient of Dr. R. N. Verney, Lyons). **a** Thorax: cardiomegaly with cardiac apex on the *left*. The stomach (*) lies beneath the right hemidiaphragm. **b** Sagittal scan of the left upper quadrant. Multiple independent splenules (*); no spleen on the *left*. **c** Angiography: opacification of the splenic artery *(arrow)*. Corresponding to situs inversus

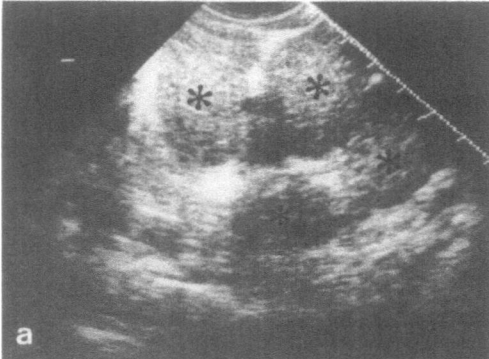

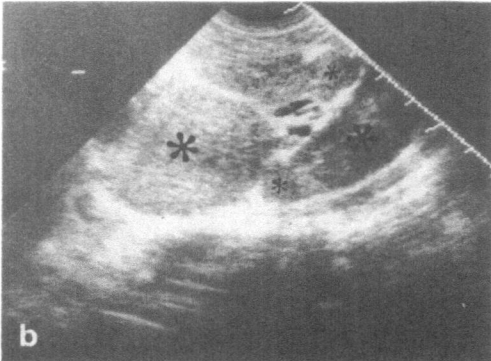

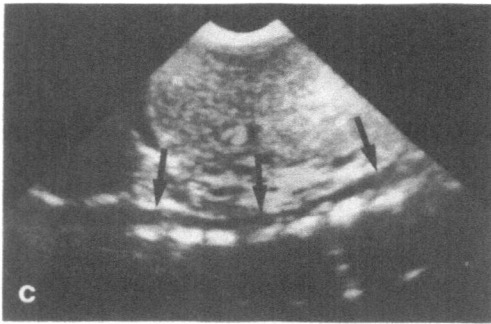

Fig. 2.5 a–c. Example of left polysplenia in a 2-year-old child with atresia of the bile ducts (corrected by surgery) and an azygos continuation of the inferior vena cava. **a** Longitudinal scan. **b** Transverse scan of the left upper quadrant. Presence of multiple rounded splenic nodules (*). **c** Longitudinal scan of the right upper quadrant. The inferior vena cava has a very posterior course *(arrows)* and terminates in the azygos vein (not seen on this scan)

Ultrasound diagnosis of the azygos continuation is relatively easy, especially on longitudinal scans: a large vein will be visualized far posterior to the diaphragm. The suprahepatic veins drain into the right atrium (Garris et al. 1980; Train et al. 1980).

2.3.3.2 Pulmonary Veins

Nearly 50% of patients have anomalous pulmonary venous drainage: the right pulmonary veins enter the right atrium while the left pulmonary veins enter the left atrium. Both pairs of pulmonary veins are distinctly separated by a ridge.

2.3.3.3 Great Vessels

Transposition of the great vessels and pulmonary atresia or stenosis are not very common (respectively 17% and 12% of cases).

2.3.3.4 Heart

The cardiac apex is located on the right in 37% of cases. The atria have the morphology of a left atrium (left atrial isomerism). The atrial septum proper is normal, but nearly 50% of patients have true atrial septal defects. The heart generally has two ventricles (90% of cases).

2.4 Wandering Spleen

Wandering spleen designates a condition in which there is loss of contact between the convex superior surface of the spleen and the concave inferior surface of the left hemidiaphragm. The condition is relatively infrequent: 97 cases were collected by Abell (1933) between 1885 and 1933. Some 60 additional cases were reported between 1960 and 1985 (Tran-Minh et al. 1984). Wandering spleen accounts for 2%–3% of all splenectomies (Gordon et al. 1977). The condition can be diagnosed at any age, in newborns as well as in elderly individuals, but most reports concern adults between 20 and 40 years old (Abell

1933). Female predominance is marked (over 90% of cases; Abell 1933). Twenty-two pediatric cases were reported between 1960 and 1985 (Barki and Bar-Ziv 1984; Broker et al. 1975, 1978; Carswell 1974; Colnet et al. 1984; Gordon et al. 1977; Martin et al. 1965; Muckmel et al. 1978; Shende et al. 1976; Stringel et al. 1982).

2.4.1 Causative Factors

Abnormal splenic mobility may be due to congenital causes and/or acquired factors (Fig. 2.6).

2.4.1.1 Congenital Causes

Literature reports mention at least four congenital causes of wandering spleen: defective splenic fixation; excessively long splenic pedicle; laxity of supporting ligaments; and particular conformation of the abdominal cavity.

Normally, the spleen is held in position by both ligaments and the pressure of contiguous organs (Gordon et al. 1977). These supporting structures include:

- The lienorenal ligament, which invests the splenic vessels and is essential for attachment of the spleen to the posterior wall
- The gastrolienal ligament, which connects the splenic hilus to the greater curvature of the stomach
- The phrenicocolic ligament ("sustentaculum lienis"), which connects the splenic flexure to the left hemidiaphragm, and serves as a sling supporting the lower pole of the spleen
- More secondary, inconstant adhesions such as the splenocolic ligament and the splenophrenic ligament

The lienorenal ligament and the gastrolienal ligament arise from the dorsal mesogastrium. The posterior investment of the left reflection of this mesentery attaches the tail of the pancreas to the retroperitoneum and in particular to the anterior surface of the left kidney. Splenic anchorage usually occurs at this point. If attachment of the posterior mesogastrium is incomplete or fails to occur (Fig. 2.6), and de-

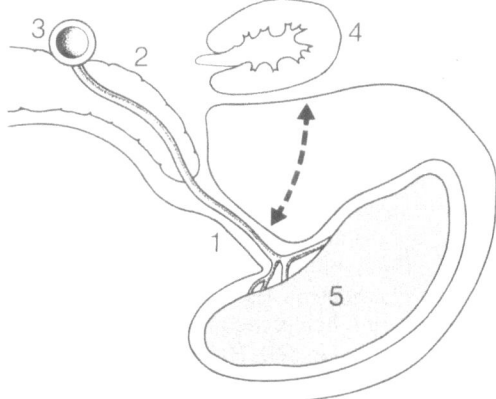

Fig. 2.6. Wandering spleen. Defective insertion of the left leaflet of the posterior mesogastrium *(1)* permits excessive mobility of the spleen *(5)* on its pedicle. The tail of the pancreas *(2)* follows the movements of the spleen. *3,* aorta; *4,* left kidney

velopmental anomalies also occur in attachment of the left colon, the spleen can move to any part of the abdomen: left iliac fossa (Atlas et al. 1985; Broker et al. 1975), the periumbilical region (Colnet et al. 1984), the pelvis (Agee et al. 1985), or even the right iliac fossa (Cross 1974; Tran-Minh et al. 1984). The spleen can also migrate into the thorax after eventration of the left diaphragm. The tail of the pancreas follows the movements of the spleen, and more precisely the splenic hilus.

Excessive splenic mobility alone can explain subsequent stretching and elongation of the vascular pedicle, although there have been reports of truly abnormally long pedicles (Abell 1933). Congenital hyperlaxity of the ligaments, and especially the phrenicocolic ligament, is another predisposing factor, as described in children with prune belly syndrome (Tait and Young 1985).

The conformation of the abdominal cavity itself has also been incriminated. For Abell (1933), "when the area between the intercostochondral arches is materially diminished while the paravertebral niches are definitely shallower ... the intra-abdominal pressure is diverted from its normal direction and prolapse occurs." In reporting on 97 cases of wandering spleen, Abell (1933) described 25 of the individuals as being of very thin or asthenic build.

2.4.1.2 Acquired Causes

Several factors predisposing to wandering spleen have been cited:

- Increase in the weight of the spleen: in the series of Abell (1933), 8 of 53 surgically resected spleens weighed 200–500 g; the other 45 organs all weighed over 500 g (the average normal adult spleen weighs 225 g). Portal hypertension (Bosniak and Byck 1960), congenital hemolytic anemia (Gordon et al. 1977; Hunter and Haber 1977), idiopathic purpura (Atlas et al. 1985), and various parasitoses (especially in endemic regions) can also cause splenomegaly.
- Relaxation of the abdominal wall and ligaments, particularly in multiparous women. Wandering spleen and its main complication, volvulus, have been encountered both during and after pregnancy (Abell 1933; Agee et al. 1985; McClain and Lebherz 1967; Miller 1975).
- A history of trauma has been implicated, although the exact mechanism remains unclear (Abell 1933).
- Gastric dilatation in the newborn can displace the spleen inferiorly: the organ is then visualized as a pseudotumor (Gordon et al. 1977; Vick et al. 1985).

For Abell (1933), at least two factors (congenital and/or acquired) always contribute to wandering spleen. Most authors, however, feel that anomalous development of the supporting ligaments in the prime cause.

2.4.2 Clinical Manifestations

Approximately two-thirds of patients give a history of abdominal pain (colicky episodes are more common than continuous pain; Abell 1933). In nearly three-fourths of cases, wandering spleen presents as an abdominal mass; pain is inconstant (Tran-Minh et al. 1984). Such smooth, hard, and oval-shaped masses are often found in the left midabdomen or the left iliac fossa; they are mobile on palpation. Occasionally, one or more characteristic notches can be detected on the anterior border during physical examination. The normal spleen is not palpable in the left upper quadrant, which gives resonance to left upper quadrant percussion. Biological tests are noncontributory, except in patients with longstanding splenomegaly.

2.4.3 Imaging Studies (Figs. 2.7 and 2.8)

2.4.3.1 Plain Abdominal Films[1]

Plain abdominal radiographs may demonstrate:

- A central abdominal mass or left flank mass related to the lower aspect of the left kidney. These oval masses have a smooth contour; on rare occasions a notched border is visible. The mass tends to descend lower in the body when the patient is examined erect.
- Excessive gas-filled loops of bowel in the left upper quadrant; a double air image is created by upwards and outwards displacement of the greater curvature of the stomach, which lies above the left colic flexure.
- Nonvisualization of the spleen in its normal position under the left hemidiaphragm.

---

[1] See Bosniak and Byck 1960; Broker et al. 1975; Colnet et al. 1984; Gordon et al. 1977; Sheflin et al. 1984.

Fig. 2.7 a–d *(above).* Uncomplicated wandering ▶ spleen in a 13-year-old boy presenting with a solitary mass in the left upper quadrant. **a** Longitudinal scan of the right upper quadrant. Homogeneous soft tissue mass *(M)* independent (⇕) from the liver *(F)* and the right kidney *(R)* with the characteristics of a spleen. No spleen on the left. **b** Celiac arteriogram; 180° rotation of the splenic artery to the right *(arrow).* The hepatic artery (↔) is normal. **c** Spleno-portal venous return. Notice the angulation of the splenic vein *(arrow)* with the portal trunk (↔). **d** Postoperative sonogram, after splenopexy. The spleen *(R)* is now in a normal position with respect to the left kidney *(RG)*

Fig. 2.8 a, b *(below).* Wandering spleen in the left periumbilical region (courtesy of Dr. Garel). **a** Longitudinal scan along the long axis of the spleen. Note the good visibility of the hilus *(arrow).* **b** Transverse scan. Note the very medial location of the spleen with respect to the aorta *(arrow)* and the spine (↔)

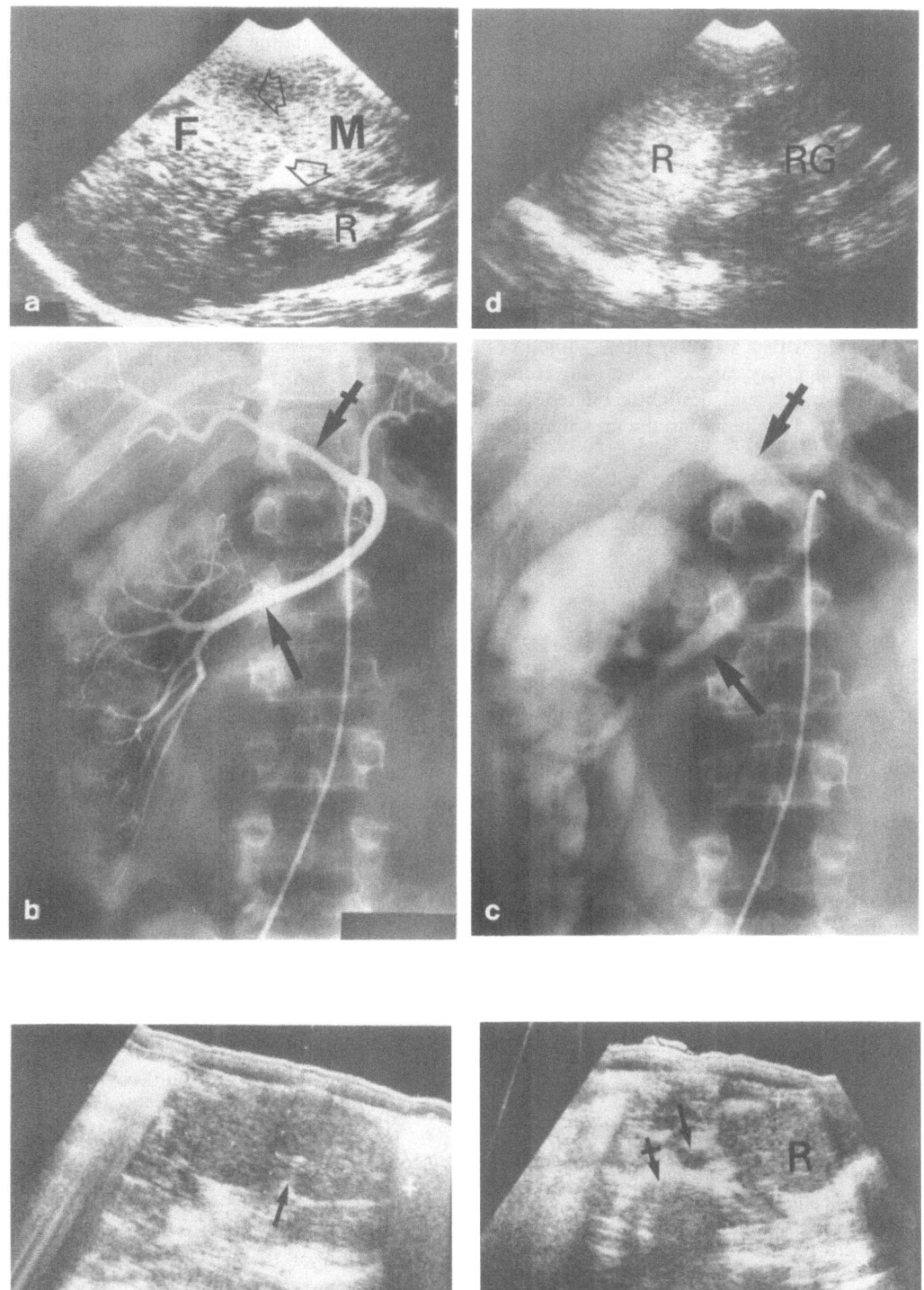

2.4.3.2 Ultrasonography[2]

The sonographic patterns of wandering spleen include:

- A solid left prerenal abdominal mass; occasionally the mass is located on the right or lies in the pelvis, behind the bladder, and displaces the uterus. Exceptionally, the mass is in direct contact with the anterior abdominal wall.
- A mass with a homogeneous solid echo pattern, without posterior reinforcement.
- A mass with a vascular hilus; sometimes a tortuous artery can be seen arising from the celiac trunk, and a slightly dilated vein is visualized draining into the mesentericoportal trunk.
- Nonvisualization of the normal spleen in the left upper quadrant.
- The tail of the pancreas presents an anterior concavity.

2.4.3.3 Scintigraphy[3]

Radioisotope scanning is the technique used most often for definitive diagnosis and the surveillance of wandering spleen, complicated or not. With the patient in the supine position, the tracer (usually ^{99m}Tc-sulfur colloid) is injected intravenously: the product accumulates in both the liver and in an oval mass located lower and more laterally than the normal spleen, which is absent from the left upper quadrant. In most cases, the long axis of a wandering spleen is oriented upwards and outwards; occasionally it is transverse. Splenic mobility can be best analyzed by having the patient change from a lying down to an erect position during scanning.

Radionuclide scanning can give false negative errors or misleading results. Use of spleen-specific tracers such as ^{51}Cr-tagged red cells can provide the correct diagnosis. Exceptionally, a direct intraarterial route is used for tracer administration.

2.4.3.4 Computed Tomography

CT can advantageously replace scintigraphy by demonstrating the absence of the spleen in the left upper quadrant, the exact location of the ectopic spleen, and the nature of its vascular pedicle and parenchyma after intravenous contrast medium injection.

2.4.3.5 Other Radiologic Techniques

When wandering spleen is suspected from the outset, the techniques listed below no longer have any indications. In other cases, they can demonstrate signs suggestive of the diagnosis.

Upper gastrointestinal series (Dublin and Rosenquist 1976; Gordon et al. 1977; Lee et al. 1979):

- Extrinsic medial compression of the greater curvature of the stomach and the small bowel
- Longitudinal rotation and elevation of the stomach
- Diverticular appearance of the greater curvature of the stomach (less frequent)

Barium enema (Gordon et al. 1977; McArdle 1980; Smulewicz and Clemett 1975):

- Anterior, medial, and inferior displacement of the true splenic flexure
- An extrinsic band-like impression on the ascending colon, near the splenic flexure
- A twisted image near the splenic flexure

Intravenous urography (Gordon et al. 1977):

- Abdominal mass lying near the inferior pole of the left kidney
- Elevation of the left kidney (inferior displacement is less common)
- Absence of the flat surface on the superoexternal aspect of the left kidney and absence of the left inferoexternal hump

---

[2] See Agee et al. 1985; Atlas et al. 1985; Barki and Bar-Ziv 1984; Colnet et al. 1984; Hunter and Haber 1977; Lee et al. 1979; McArdle 1980; Miller 1975; Sheflin et al. 1984; Tait and Young 1985.

[3] See Agee et al. 1985; Atlas et al. 1985; Barki and Bar-Ziv 1984; Broker et al. 1975; Colnet et al. 1984; Dublin and Rosenquist 1976; Gordon et al. 1977; Hatfield et al. 1976; Hunter and Haber 1977; Isikoff et al. 1977; Lee et al. 1979; McArdle 1980; Rosenthall et al. 1974; Sheflin et al. 1984; Tait and Young 1985; Toback et al. 1984.

- Anteroposterior compression of the ureters, above the pelvic brim: no lateral ureteral displacement
- Occasionally, marked dilatation of the left ureter and renal pelves and calices

Angiography (Gordon et al. 1977; Hatfield et al. 1976; Levasseur et al. 1973; McArdle 1980; Sheflin et al. 1984; Shende et al. 1976; Smulewicz and Clemett 1971). Intravenous abdominal aortography or, better yet, selective injection into the celiac artery can demonstrate:

- An elongated, slightly tortuous or straight splenic artery descending vertically to the left of the spine; occasionally, the splenic artery turns towards the right iliac fossa or the right upper quadrant.
- Recurrent course of the vessels of the tail of the pancreas.
- Homogeneous appearance of the splenic parenchyma.
- Ascending course of the splenic vein towards the portal vein (superomedially and to the left).

Splenoportography has been used occasionally for the workup of patients with portal hypertension; partial stenosis of the splenic vein may be visualized.

2.4.4 Treatment of Uncomplicated Wandering Spleen

A wandering spleen can remain totally asymptomatic: the patient may merely be aware of an abdominal mass or an enlarged spleen, possibly for several years. Once diagnosed, wandering spleen warrants surgery to avoid possible complications (torsion of the pedicle, acute colic occlusion by adhesions, progressive portal hypertension, formation of intrasplenic pseudocysts). Nonoperative management is reserved for very elderly individuals and patients with progressive neoplastic disease (Gordon et al. 1977; Lee et al. 1979; Tait and Young 1985).

Splenectomy, the most common procedure, eliminates the risks of torsion or splenic rupture due to trauma, which is especially elevated in pregnant women. However, splenectomy has been criticized for reducing the patient's resistance to infections. While this is true in very young infants, it is less so in older children, adolescents, and adults. *Splenopexy* has the advantage of conserving the functional splenic tissue. The renewed interest in this once nearly abandonned technique is due to several technical improvements (special sutures, biological adhesives, etc.). The risk of recurrence after splenopexy is very low. Ultrasonography can usefully monitor splenic repositioning and the organ's echo pattern, but actual splenic function can be evaluated only by radionuclide scanning.

2.4.5 Torsion of the Splenic Pedicle

The most frequent and most serious complication of wandering spleen is volvulus or torsion of the spleen, defined as twisting of the organ on its pedicle in one or more clockwise or counterclockwise turns – up to 8 turns have been reported (Fig. 2.9, p. 26; Abell 1933; Broker et al. 1978; Carswell 1974; Cross 1974; DeBartolo et al. 1973; Dublin and Rosenquist 1976; Gordon et al. 1977; Lee et al. 1979; McArdle 1980; McClain and Lebherz 1967; Martin et al. 1965; Miller 1975; Muckmel et al. 1978; Rosenthall et al. 1974; Sheflin et al. 1984; Shende et al. 1976; Smulewicz and Clemett 1975).

Torsion of the splenic pedicle leads to progressively severe vascular compromise: venous occlusion, passive congestion, arterial occlusion, parenchymal ischemia with increased congestion, hemorrhagic infarction, and sometimes necrosis or abscess formation (Shende 1976).

2.4.5.1 Subacute and Chronic Torsion

The circulatory damage caused by subacute and chronic torsion is reversible, and never progresses beyond passive congestion. Detorsion can occur spontaneously, although there is a risk of splenomegaly at long term. Perisplenic adhesions, fibrous scarring due to old localized infarction in the hilus and around the spleen, and increased venous circulation are all frequent.

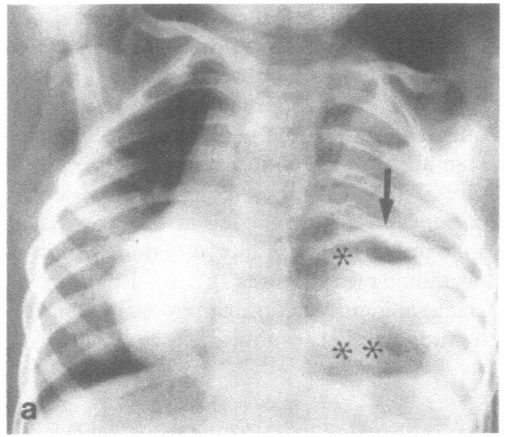

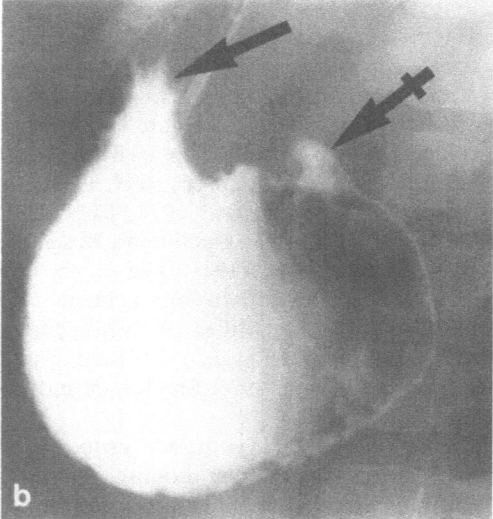

Fig. 2.9 a, b. Torsion of the spleen with left diaphragmatic eventration. This 20-month-old child presented a painful acute abdomen of sudden onset with vomiting (+++). Ultrasonography was not performed. **a** Thorax. Elevation of the left hemidiaphragm *(arrow)*. The left colic flexure (*) is abnormally high and lies medial to the stomach (**). **b** Lateral view of an upper gastrointestinal study: the greater curvature of the stomach *(arrow)* is twisted owing to torsion of the spleen (pylorus; ↦)

2.4.5.2 Acute Torsion

Acute torsion of the splenic pedicle causes occlusion of the splenic artery and vein; involvement of just one of these vessels is rare. The hemorrhagic infarction accompanying acute torsion can lead secondarily to abscess formation. Involvement of the tail of the pancreas in the twisted pedicle can result in hemorrhagic necrosis (Shende 1976).

2.4.5.3 Causative Factors

Torsion of the splenic pedicle implicates the same predisposing factors as wandering spleen in general: splenomegaly, pregnancy or the postpartum period, and trauma. For Woodward (1967), however, a developmental anomaly (incomplete fusion of the mesogastrium posteriorly) is the prime cause of increased splenic mobility, with laxity of the gastrosplenic ligament being only one of several precipitating factors.

2.4.5.4 Clinical Manifestations

Presenting symptoms are typical of acute abdomen: severe, progressive abdominal pain of sudden onset accompanied by nausea and vomiting. Physical examination may elicit three characteristic findings (Carswell 1974): palpation of an ovoid abdominal mass with a notched border; easy, nonpainful movement of this mass towards the left upper quadrant but limited, painful movement in other directions; resonance to percussion in the left upper quadrant. Peripheral blood smears will reveal leukocytosis and thrombocytosis. The presence of deformed erythrocytes and Howell-Jolly bodies in the red blood cells reflects functional asplenia.

2.4.5.5 Radiologic Signs

Plain abdominal films (McClain and Lebherz 1967; Martin et al. 1965):

– Ovoid midabdominal mass with contours clearly outlined by gas; a notched border is pathognomonic for a splenic mass.

- Location of the gastric air bubble entirely under the left hemidiaphragm.
- Medial displacement of the left colic flexure.
- Intestinal ileus.

Ultrasonography (McArdle 1980; Muckmel et al. 1978; Sheflin et al. 1984):

- Signs of wandering spleen (cf. Section 2.4.3.2)
- Intraperitoneal fluid
- An enlarged, inhomogeneous pancreas, when the tail of this organ is involved in splenic torsion

Radioisotope scanning is rarely performed in an emergency setting, but will demonstrate total absence of tracer accumulation by the spleen. Direct intraarterial injection of the radionuclide sometimes permits detection of slight fixation, probably as the result of partial spontaneous detorsion of the pedicle. The clinical picture of acute abdomen makes it possible to rule out the other causes of functional asplenia detected by scintigraphy: sickle-cell anemia, Thorotrast deposition, reticulum cell sarcoma, or intrathoracic transposition of the spleen (Rosenthall et al. 1974).

Celiac angiography may visualize abrupt, severe stenosis of the splenic artery. Complete or partial persistent uptake by the splenic parenchyma is indicative of focal infarction. The splenic vein is not demonstrated.

2.4.5.6 Treatment

Emergency treatment generally consists in splenectomy. The mortality rate ranges from 20%–50%. Splenopexy is sometimes performed in children if the organ appears viable and was healthy prior to torsion. Postoperative radioisotope scanning allows detection of accessory spleens.

2.5 Splenogonadal Fusion

Splenogonadal fusion is a very rare congenital malformation resulting from abnormal fusion of the splenic and gonadal anlagen arising from the mesonephros (Fig. 2.10). Male pre-

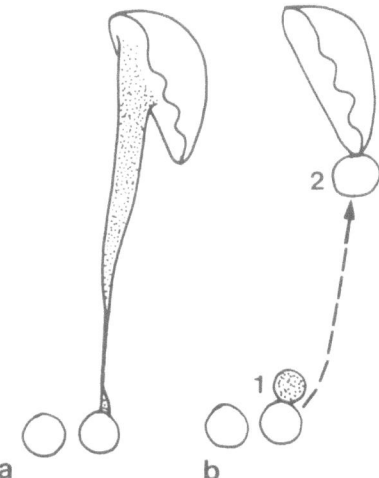

Fig. 2.10 a, b. Splenogonadal fusion. **a** Continuous splenogonadal fusion with a fibrous and/or tissular connecting cord between the spleen and the left testicle. **b** Discontinuous splenogonadal fusion: *1*, solitary splenic nodule attached to the testicle; *2*, attachment of an ectopic testicle to the spleen (less common)

dominance is marked (approximately 95% of cases; Given and Guiney 1978; Watson 1968). The defect is seen almost exclusively in Caucasian individuals, and is diagnosed slightly more often in children than in adults.

2.5.1 Anatomic Classification

Putschar and Manion (1956b) defined two types of splenogonadal fusion: continuous and discontinuous.

2.5.1.1 Continuous Splenogonadal Fusion

In individuals with continuous splenogonadal fusion, the most frequent form, a cord of tissue connects the regular spleen with the left testicle or, less often, with the epididymis, ovary, or mesovarium. There has been only one report of splenogonal fusion involving the right gonadal structures. Ranging in diameter from several millimeters to one centimeter, this cord usually arises from the superior pole of the spleen. It can also arise from the inferior pole, the hilus or the anterior border. The shape of this connecting structure varies from a tapered, tubular band to a cord with outgrowths of splenic tissue at its origin and/or point of termination.

Histologically, the connecting cord may consist of normal splenic tissue, of disorganized splenic tissue, or of fibrous tissue (especially in the lower third). Splenic nodules may be present along the cord or around the spleen. The cord often contains an autonomous arteriovenous pedicle.

The lower point of attachment is usually the superior or inferior pole of the left testicle. The splenic and gonadal tissues are separated by a more or less thick band of fibrous tissue. Selective resection with preservation of the testicle depends on whether or not the ectopic splenic tissue is covered by the tunica vaginalis.

2.5.1.2 Discontinuous Splenogonadal Fusion

Discontinuous splenogonadal fusion can be considered a particular variant of accessory spleen as there is no anatomic connection between the regular and the ectopic spleens (Fig. 2.11, p. 29). Most cases involve a single testicular nodule ranging in size from 4–5 cm; occasionally there are two or three such nodules. Only the left side is affected.

2.5.2 Associated Anomalies

Congenital left inguinal hernia is almost constant (Tonkin and Tonkin 1982), and the left testicle is frequently mobile or ectopic (Tsingoglou and Wilkinson 1976). The relative frequency of associated micrognathia and limb anomalies (complete or incomplete absence of one or more members or segments of members) led to designation of this malformation complex as Putschar's syndrome (Putschar and Manion 1956a, b). Associations with cleft soft palate, microgastria (Mandell et al. 1983), and cardiovascular defects have also been reported.

2.5.3 Pathogenesis

The spleen forms in the left dorsal mesogastrium during the 5th week in the 8–10 mm embryo. It consists of several small masses which fuse secondarily. The splenic anlage is in close apposition to the mesonephros and the gonadal anlagen before the latter descend during the 8th week. For some unknown reason, fusion occurs during the 5th and 8th weeks of gestation; an inflammatory process has been suggested. Discontinuous splenogonadal fusion probably is the result of one or more splenic buds that develop separately from the main spleen.

2.5.4 Circumstances of Detection

Most cases of splenogonadal fusion are discovered at operation for left inguinal hernia, during testicular exploration for cryptorchidism or a scrotal mass, or at autopsy. Certain patients, however, may present various local symptoms: pain, discomfort and swelling of the scrotum after long marches (soldiers) or physical exercise in general; so-called recurrent epididymo-orchitis; a mass in the left testicle present since birth; scrotal enlargement during malarial attacks or systemic infections. Other accompanying signs not directly localized to the inguinal region or testicle include chronic occlusion of the large intestine (Hines and Eggum 1961), a combination of multiple malformations, and menorrhagia (Tsingoglou and Wilkinson 1976).

2.5.5 Differential Diagnosis

Positive diagnosis of splenogonadal fusion is extremely rare before surgery or autopsy. The major differential diagnoses for a mass in the left testicle include: inguinal hernia with the presence of omentum, a third testicle, testicular tumor, thrombosis of the spermatic vessels, tuberculous or nonspecific epididymo-orchitis, diffuse lymphangioma of the spermatic cord, splenosis nodule (Bennett-Jones and St Hill 1952; Sieber 1969).

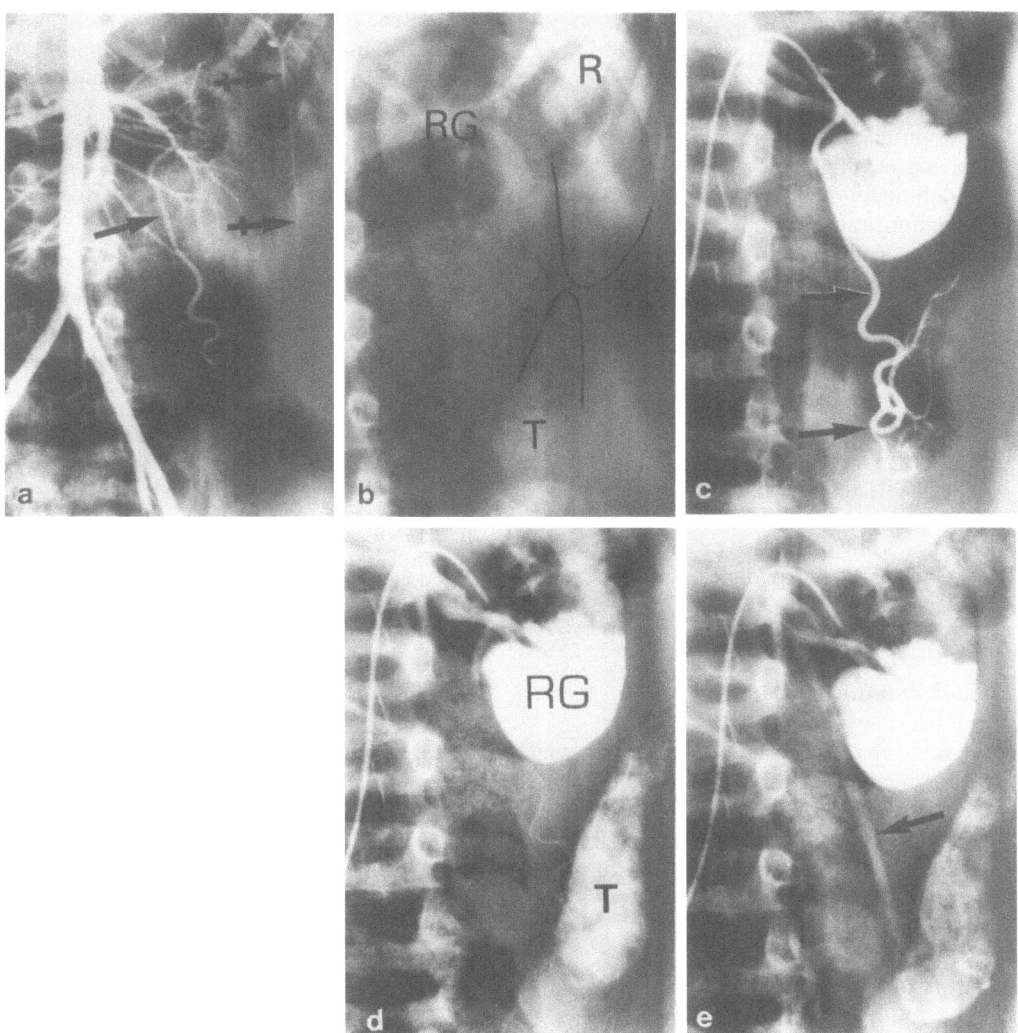

Fig. 2.11 a–e. Discontinuous splenogonadal fusion with an ectopic testicle in a 4-year-old child hospitalized for genital examinations (courtesy of Prof. M. Hassan). **a** Abdominal aortography. Abnormal spermatic pedicle *(arrow)* arising from the left inferior polar renal artery. Note the long splenic artery (↔). **b** Aortography, late phase. The inferior pole of the spleen *(R)* and the superior pole of the ectopic testicle *(T)* are in contact. *RG,* left kidney. **c** Selective arteriography: tortuous spermatic artery *(arrow)*. **d** Soft tissue phase showing the ectopic left testicle *(T)* near the left kidney *(RG)*. **e** Spermatic venous return *(arrow)* into the left renal vein

2.5.6 *Imaging Studies*

2.5.6.1 *Radionuclide Scanning*

^{99m}Tc-sulfur colloid radionuclide scanning (McLean et al. 1981; Mandell et al. 1983) is the definitive diagnostic examination which will demonstrate the main spleen in its normal anatomic position and one or more ectopic nodules also taking up the tracer. In one very favorable case, the upper portion of the cord was visualized (McLean et al. 1981).

2.5.6.2 *Arteriography*

Owing to its invasive nature, arteriography is not commonly performed. However, it may accurately localize one or more abnormal splenic or testicular pedicles and their venous drainage system (Fig. 2.11).

2.5.6.3 *Ultrasonography*

Although we are unaware of any case in which splenogonadal fusion has been diagnosed sonographically, it is technically feasible. The sonographer should keep this possibility in mind when examining the scrotum of a child with multiple birth defects.

2.5.6.4 *Treatment*

Continuous splenogonadal fusion is treated by resection of the cord; extemporaneous histologic examination will confirm the splenic nature of the resected tissue. Discontinuous splenogonadal fusion is treated either by en bloc resection (when the splenic nodule and the testicle are both covered by the tunica vaginalis) or by selective exeresis of the splenic nodule.

2.6 Conclusion

Ultrasonography should be the first imaging technique used for positive diagnosis of splenic anomalies and associated malformations (especially abdominal and cardiovascu-lar defects). Sonographic examination is particularly indicated for children. Computed tomography and radioisotope scanning can be utilized as second stage procedures. If these imaging studies fail to provide a clear diagnosis or complementary preoperative data is desirable, angiography can then be performed.

2.7 References

Abell I (1933) Wandering spleen with torsion of the pedicle. Ann Surg 98: 722–735
Agee JH, Crepps LF, Layton M (1985) Wandering pelvic spleen. J Clin Ultrasound 13: 145–146
Atlas SW, Rochester D, Panella JS, Larson R (1985) The utility of ultrasound in the diagnosis of wandering abdominal viscera. J Clin Ultrasound 13: 275–277
Barki Y, Bar-Ziv J (1984) Wandering spleen in two children. The role of ultrasonic diagnosis. Br J Radiol 57: 267–270
Bennett-Jones MJ, St Hill CA (1952) Accessory spleen in the scrotum. Br J Surg 40: 259–262
Bosniak MA, Byck W (1960) Wandering spleen diagnosed preoperatively by intravenous aortography. AJR 84: 898–901
Broker FHL, Khettry J, Filler RM, Treves S (1975) Splenic torsion and accessory spleen: a scintigraphic demonstration. J Pediatr Surg 10: 913–915
Broker FHL, Fellows K, Treves S (1978) Wandering spleen in three children. Pediatr Radiol 6: 211–214
Carswell JW (1974) Wandering spleen: 11 cases from Uganda. Br J Surg 61: 495–497
Chandra RS (1974) Biliary atresia and other structural anomalies in the congenital polysplenia syndrome. J Pediatr 85: 649–655
Colnet H, Diard F, Calabet A, Broussin B, Hehunstre JP (1984) La rate errante. A propos d'une observation chez un enfant de 4 ans. Arch Fr Pediatr 41: 139–141
Cross AB (1974) Diagnostic clue to acute splenic torsion in the tropics. Br Med J 3: 564–566
Curet P, Dyart J, Tucat G, Chartrain J, Grellet J (1980) Polysplénie sans anomalie cardiaque patente. Un cas étudié par artériographie superselective. J Radiol 61: 65–68
DeBartolo HM Jr, van Heerden JA, Lynn HB, Norris DG (1973) Torsion of the spleen: a case report. Mayo Clin Proc 48: 781–786
Dublin AB, Rosenquist CJ (1976) Case report. Diagnosis of splenic torsion: a combined radiographic approach. Br J Radiol 49: 1045–1046
Elliott LP, Cramer GG, Amplatz K (1966) The anomalous relationship of the inferior vena cava and abdominal aorta as a specific angiocardiographic sign in asplenia. Radiology 87: 859–863

Fitzer PM (1976) An approach to cardiac malposition and the heterotaxy syndrome using ^{99m}Tc sulfur colloid imaging. AJR 127: 1021–1025

Floyd GD, Nelson WP (1976) Developmental interruption of the inferior vena cava with azygos and hemiazygos substitution. Unusual radiographic features. Radiology 119: 55–57

Freedom RM (1972) The asplenia syndrome: a review of significant extracardiac structural abnormalities in 29 necropsied patients. J Pediatr 81: 1130–1133

Freedom RM, Fellows KE Jr (1973) Radiographic visceral patterns in the asplenia syndrome. Radiology 106: 387–391

Freedom RM, Treves S (1973) Splenic scintigraphy and radionuclide venography in the heterotaxy syndrome. Radiology 107: 381–386

Garris JB, Kangarloo H, Sample WF (1980) Ultrasonic diagnosis of infrahepatic interruption of the inferior vena cava with azygos (hemiazygos) continuation. Radiology 134: 179–183

Given HF, Guiney EJ (1978) Splenic-gonadal fusion. J Pediatr Surg 13: 341

Gordon DH, Burrell MI, Levin DC, Mueller CF, Becker JA (1977) Wandering spleen – the radiological and clinical spectrum. Radiology 125: 39–46

Gray SW, Skandalakis JE (1972) Embryology for surgeons. The embryological basis for the treatment of congenital defects. Saunders, Philadelphia

Haswell DM, Berrigan TJ Jr (1976) Anomalous inferior vena cava with accessory hemiazygos continuation. Radiology 119: 51–54

Hatfield PM, Clouse ME, Cady B (1976) Ectopic pelvic spleen. Arch Surg 111: 603–605

Heller RM, Dorst JP, James AE Jr, Rowe RD (1971) A useful sign in the recognition of azygos continuation of the inferior vena cava. Radiology 101: 519–522

Hines JR, Eggum PR (1961) Splenic-gonadal fusion causing bowel obstruction. Arch Surg 83: 887–889

Hunter TB, Haber K (1977) Sonographic diagnosis of a wandering spleen. AJR 129: 925–926

Isikoff MB, White DW, Diaconis JN (1977) Torsion of the wandering spleen, seen as a migratory abdominal mass. Radiology 123: 36

Kessler H, Smulewicz JJ (1973) Microgastria associated with agenesis of the spleen. Radiology 107: 393–396

Khattar HF, Petitclerc R, Gilbert G, Aerichide N, Bourassa M (1972) Le syndrome de polysplénie et les malformations cardiaques et viscérales associées. A propos de 2 cas et revue de 46 cas de la littérature. Cœur 3: 619–635

Lee TG, Brickman FE, Satterwhite GR, Avecilla LS (1979) Ultrasound demonstration of wandering spleen. Arch Surg 114: 13–15

Levasseur JC, Mafioli C, Menanteau B (1973) Splénomégalie et ectopie de la rate. Sem Hôp Paris 49: 2697–2698

Mandell GA, Heyman S, Alavi A, Ziegler MM (1983) A case of microgastria in association with splenic-gonadal fusion. Pediatr Radiol 13: 95–98

Martin JP, Chamlou I, Buzyn E (1965) Un cas de torsion aiguë de la rate chez un nourisson de 6 mois. Ann Chir Inf 6: 149–152

McArdle C (1980) Case of the winter season: torsion of a wandering spleen. Sem Roentgenol 15: 7–8

McClain GH, Lebherz TB (1967) Radiographic evidence of splenic torsion: report of a case. Obst Gyn 29: 475–478

McLean GK, Alavi A, Ziegler MM, Pollack HM, Duckett JW (1981) Splenic-gonadal fusion: identification by radionuclide scanning. J Pediatr Surg 16: 649–651

Miller EI (1975) Wandering spleen and pregnancy: case report. J Clin Ultrasound 3: 281–282

Muckmel E, Zer M, Dintsman M (1978) Wandering spleen with torsion of pedicle in a child presenting as an intermittently appearing abdominal mass. J Pediatr Surg 13: 127–128

Putschar WGJ, Manion WC (1956a) Congenital absence of the spleen and associated anomalies. Am J Clin Pathol 26: 429–470

Putschar WGJ, Manion WC (1956b) Splenic-gonadal fusion. Am J Pathol 32: 15–33

Randall PA, Moller JH, Amplatz K (1973) The spleen and congenital heart disease. AJR 119: 551–559

Rao BK, Shore RM, Lieberman KM, Polcyn RE (1982) Dual radiopharmaceutical imaging in congenital asplenia syndrome. Radiology 145: 805–810

Rose V, Izukawa T, Moës CAF (1975) Syndromes of asplenia and polysplenia. A review of cardiac and non-cardiac malformations in 60 cases with special reference to diagnosis and prognosis. Br Heart J 37: 840–852

Rosenthall L, Lisbona R, Banerjee K (1974) A nucleographic and radioangiographic study of a patient with torsion of the spleen. Radiology 110: 427–428

Sheflin JR, Lee CM, Kretchmar KA (1984) Torsion of wandering spleen and distal pancreas. AJR 142: 100–101

Shende A, Lanzkowsky P, Becker J (1976) Torsion of a visceroptosed spleen. Am J Dis Child 130: 88–91

Sieber WK (1969) Splenotesticular cord (splenogonadal fusion) associated with inguinal hernia. J Pediatr Surg 4: 208–210

Smulewicz JJ, Clemett AR (1975) Torsion of the wandering spleen. Am J Dig Dis 20: 274–279

Soto B, Pacifico AD, Souza AS Jr, Bargeron LM Jr, Ermocilla R, Tonkin IL (1978) Identification of thoracic isomerism from the plain chest radiograph. AJR 131: 995–1002

Stringel G, Soucy P, Mercer S (1982) Torsion of the wandering spleen: splenectomy or splenopexy. J Pediatr Surg 17: 373–375

Tait NP, Young JR (1985) The wandering spleen: an ultrasonic diagnosis. J Clin Ultrasound 13: 141–144

Toback AC, Steece DM, Kaye MD (1984) Splenic torsion: an unusual cause of splenomegaly. Dig Dis Sci 29: 868–871

Tonkin ILD, Tonkin AK (1982) Visceroatrial situs abnormalities: sonographic and computed tomographic appearance. AJR 138: 509–515

Train JS, Henderson MR, Smith AP (1980) Sonographic demonstration of left-sided inferior vena cava with hemiazygos continuation. AJR 134: 1057–1059

Tran-Minh VA, Pracros JP, Deffrenne P (1984) Echographie de la rate chez l'enfant. Société Française de Radiologie, Enseignement post-universitaire, Paris

Tsingoglou S, Wilkinson AW (1976) Splenogonadal fusion. Br J Surg 63: 297–298

Van Mierop LHS, Gessner IH, Schiebler GL (1972) Asplenia and polysplenia syndrome. Birth Def 8: 74–82

Vaughan TJ, Hawkins IF Jr, Elliott LP (1971) Diagnosis of polysplenia syndrome. Radiology 101: 511–518

Vick CW, Hartenberg MA, Allen HA, Haynes JW (1985) Abdominal pseudotumor caused by gastric displacement of the spleen. Pediatr Radiol 15: 253–254

Watson RJ (1968) Splenogonadal fusion. Surgery 63: 853–858

Woodward DAK (1967) Torsion of the spleen. Am J Surg 114: 953–955

3 Splenic Trauma

M. BENOZIO

Although ultrasonography was rapidly adopted for exploration of the traumatized spleen, there are few recent reports on the actual value and limitations of such examinations. Large, homogeneous study populations are difficult to collect as the quality of sonographic investigations at a given institution can vary with time and as a function of the examiner. Many reports deal with retrospective series, but correlations with histology findings can be complicated by changing concepts concerning the indications for splenectomy (Farthmann et al. 1985; Solheim and Hoivik 1985). The introduction of gray scale equipment confirmed the utility of the technique for evaluating splenic trauma, inasmuch as hemoperitoneum could be demonstrated (Asher et al. 1976). The successive development of real-time apparatus and sector scanners saw notable improvements in the quality of sonographic images (Weill et al. 1981). By this time, ultrasonography had proven its reliability for examination of the solid abdominal organs (Amici et al. 1982; Aufschnaiter and Kofler 1983; Halbfass et al. 1981; Hauenstein et al. 1982) and had become a valid alternative to computed tomography for both adult and pediatric patients (Babcock and Kaufman 1983; Berger and Kuhn 1981; Filiatrault et al. 1984; Kaufman et al. 1984; Klels et al. 1983; Viscomi et al. 1980).

3.1 Causes and Clinical Manifestations

Among the many causes of blunt abdominal trauma, motor vehicle accidents and athletic injuries are both on the rise, in children as in adults. Falls are another common mechanism of injury, especially in attempted suicide by young individuals. Underlying disease and iatrogenic injury are other notable causes (Jones et al. 1983).

Three patterns of splenic injury have been described:

- Multiple injury patients in whom splenic trauma may be masked by a head injury, fractures of the extremities, or thoracic or retroperitoneal injury (over 50% of cases)
- Blunt trauma to the entire abdomen, with signs of intraperitoneal hemorrhage and severe hemorrhagic shock
- Trauma isolated to the splenic region or the left upper quadrant, with local or diffuse pain, nausea and vomiting, guarding, abdominal gas, pallor, quick pulse, hypotension, and pain on rectal examination.

Imaging studies have few indications for the first two categories, except for rapid ultrasound examinations at the patient's bedside. Patients with the third type of trauma, however, generally require imaging studies for proper management.

3.2 Ultrasonography of the Traumatized Spleen

When determining the indications for sonographic examination of patients who have sustained splenic injury, several points warrant consideration:

- Is ultrasonography indicated for exploration of apparently minor splenic injuries? Should it be performed when splenic trauma is merely suspected?
- Can ultrasonography help reduce the incidence of delayed splenic rupture?
- Can sonographic patterns be used to characterize lesion evolution, thereby shortening the duration of follow-up studies?
- Can sonographic findings be correlated with the histologic features of splenic lesions, thereby obviating the need for sple-

nectomy or allowing conservative management in certain cases?

3.2.1 Technique

Trauma patients have already received emergency treatment to stabilize vital signs before they are examined by a sonographer. Splenic sonography must obligatorily be preceded by a chest radiograph and a plain abdominal film. The chest X-ray will reveal any associated traumatic lesions and may indirectly suggest the existence of splenic injury: diaphragmatic tear, pleural effusion, or pulmonary hematoma. A high incidence of concomitant lower left rib fractures has been noted in adults (over 40% of cases in our experience). Plain abdominal films may disclose signs suggestive of a splenic lesion or hemoperitoneum, but are especially helpful in demonstrating signs of a hollow viscus lesion or retroperitoneal injury. Ultrasonography is always performed before diagnostic peritoneal lavage.

The advantages and limitations of linear transducers and sector scanners highlight the utility of multihead instruments. Sector scanners are probably the best model for examination.

Difficulties encountered during examination are linked to the nature of intraabdominal injuries:

- A thorough search must be made for associated lesions, in particular injury of the liver and kidneys.
- Optimum examination positions are not always possible when patients cannot be mobilized or are in pain, and parietal contact with the transducer may not be tolerated; likewise, the presence of abdominal gas can interfere with sonographic investigation.
- Sonograms must always be interpreted with reference to the clinical context.

3.2.2 Sonographic Features of Splenic Lesions

3.2.2.1 Free Intraperitoneal Fluid

With the patient lying supine, the most dependent body recesses must always be examined first for the presence of free intraperitoneal fluid: Morison pouch (hepatorenal fossa), jux-

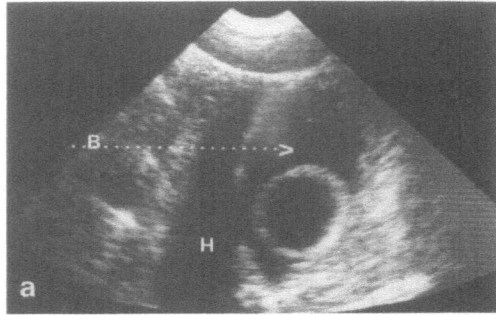
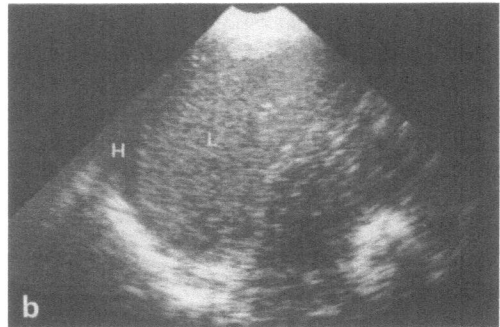

Fig. 3.1 a, b. Intraperitoneal fluid: pelvic (**a**) and perihepatic (**b**) effusions. *B*, bladder with catheter; *H*, hematoma; *L*, liver

tasplenic recess, pouch of Douglas, beneath the anterolateral abdominal wall, in the paracolic gutters (Federle and Jeffrey 1983; Hauenstein et al. 1982; Hicken et al. 1981). These sonolucent effusions appear crescent-shaped when confined in recesses; when free in the peritoneal cavity they will appear diffuse. A fluid-like image separating intestinal loops or occupying the flanks suggests abundant effusion. The rapid appearance of relatively fine echoes throughout such zones corresponds to the formation of blood clots: such patterns are particularly suggestive when located around parenchymal lesions (Fig. 3.1). From this point on, two types of evolution are possible: (a) organization or establishment, with the appearance of septations indicative of fibrin formation and sedimentation, or (b) liquefaction, possibly leading to the formation of true traumatic pseudocysts. In both cases, echo patterns can vary both with time and from one point of a lesion to another. Abscess formation is demonstrated as a lesion containing multiple fine hyperechoic images with posterior acoustic shadowing, corresponding to the presence of intralesion gas.

While the sonographic features mentioned above are often diagnostic, echo patterns visualized shortly after trauma has occurred can be difficult to interpret. A small effusion detected in the absence of any relevant clinical context may merely be a physiological occurrence. Patients must be examined in several positions to determine whether an effusion is present between the spleen and left kidney: displacement of the fluid image on sonograms will confirm injury. In certain cases, the seminal vesicles can be visualized within an extensive retrovesical effusion.

Occasionally, ultrasonography allows quantitative evaluation of intraperitoneal effusions, which can be classed as mild, moderate, or severe. Such qualitative assessment may be preferable to attempts to measure the thickness of effusions in the subhepatic region, an area where effusions less than 0.5 cm thick usually correspond to less than 500 ml (Hauenstein et al. 1982).

Before discussing actual splenic lesions, it must be remembered that hemoperitoneum in a patient with abdominal injuries only suggests splenic trauma. All of the solid viscera and other structures amenable to ultrasonography must be examined, because 10%–20% of patients have associated injuries of the liver, kidneys, retroperitoneal walls, digestive tract, or large vessels, or rupture of the left hemidiaphragm (Aufschnaiter and Kofler 1983; Halbfass et al. 1981; Kaufman et al. 1984; Weill et al. 1981). Finally, complete absence of any effusion is also possible, namely in cases of nonruptured subcapsular splenic hematoma.

3.2.2.2 Intrasplenic Lesions

Owing to the varied nature of splenic lesions, their evolutionary course, and the frequency of other associated injuries, correlation of sonographic features with histopathologic data is rarely perfect. This is true even after laparotomy or splenectomy, as these procedures are often performed some time after the ultrasound examination (Johnson et al. 1981; Jones et al. 1983; Kuhn et al. 1983; Schulz and Willi

1983; van Sonnenberg et al. 1983; Vergé-Garret et al. 1983; Wilson et al. 1978).

Typical sonographic anomalies detected in patients with splenic trauma include:

- Splenic enlargement with hyperechoic internal defects indicating contusions of the pulp (Fig. 3.2)
- Anechoic images representing intrasplenic hematomas at varying stages of organization (Fig. 3.3)
- Curved anechoic peripheral lesions corresponding to subcapsular hematomas (Fig. 3.4)
- One or more linear anechoic intrasplenic defects indicative of fracture(s) (Fig. 3.5)

The importance of several nonspecific signs must also be emphasized:

- Splenomegaly (diameter over 10 cm measured on the axillary line)
- Irregular splenic margins (Fig. 3.6)
- Loss of large vessel images at the hilus

Examination must also take into account several other possibilities:

- Lesions limited to discretely inhomogeneous splenomegaly (Fig. 3.7).
- In approximately 10% of patients the spleen is not visualized at all, or is only poorly imaged: this is an important fact to be kept in mind.
- Splenic sonograms may appear normal, yet be associated with a peritoneal fluid effusion.

Table 3.1 summarizes possible echo pattern combinations in cases where ultrasound examination is considered complete or at least satisfactory (approximately 90% of cases). The hemorrhagic nature of intraperitoneal fluid can be confirmed by diagnostic peritoneal lavage: this procedure is primarily indicated for spleens that appear sonographically normal or have been insufficiently explored by ultrasound.

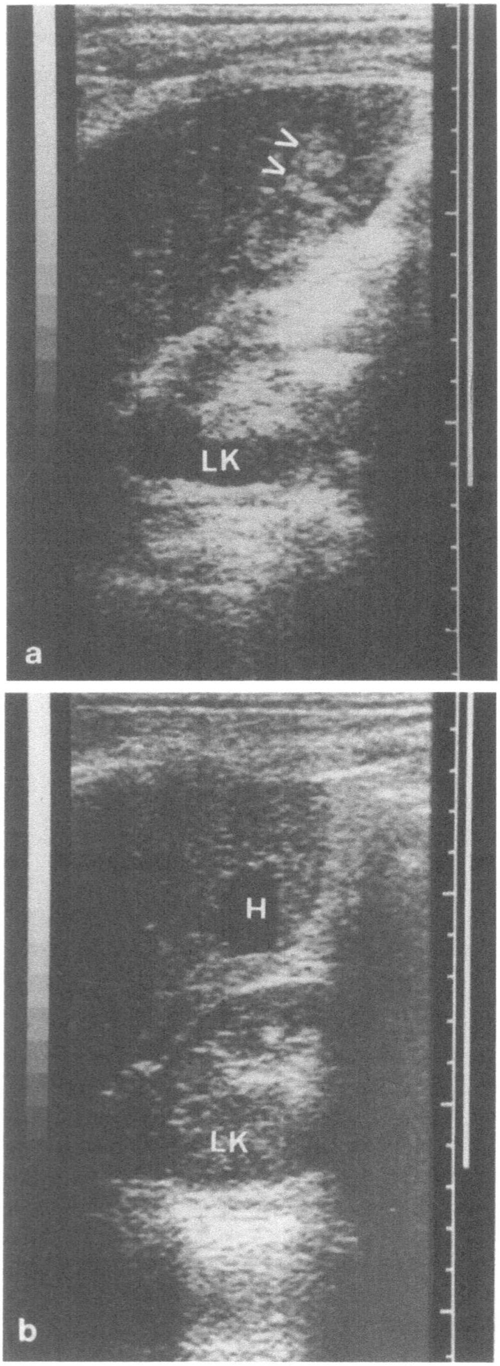

Fig. 3.2 a, b.   Multiple splenic injuries: hyperechoic contusion *(arrows)* (a) and small transsonic hematomas *(H)* (b). *LK*, left kidney

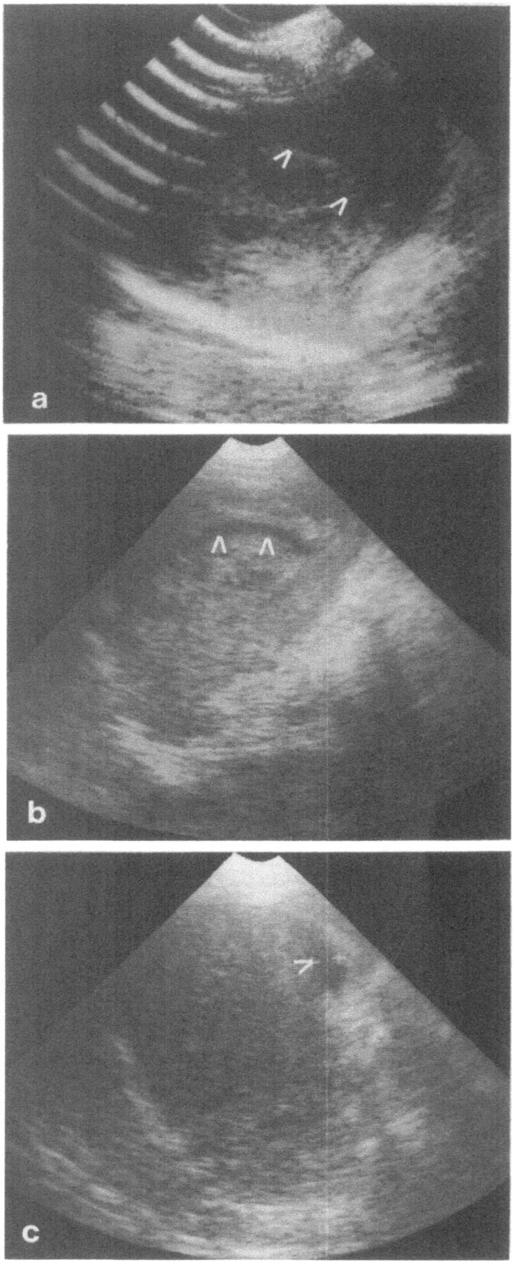

Fig. 3.3 a–c.   Three examples of intrasplenic hematoma *(arrows)*

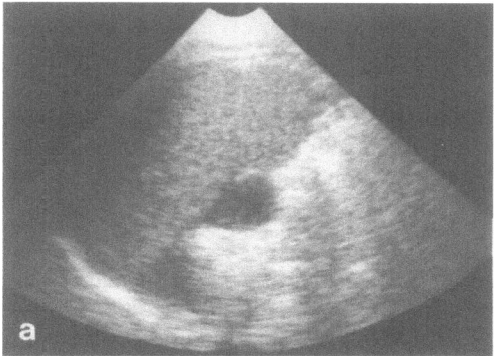

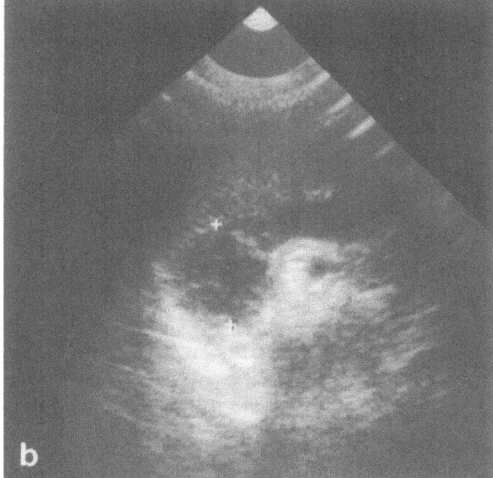

Fig. 3.4a, b. Rounded, juxtahilar subcapsular hematoma (day 1) (**a**) and stable appearance on day 20 (**b**); 2 cm between the two *crosses*

Table 3.1. Sonographic detection of splenic anomalies and effusion in connection with 84 surgically proven splenic lesions

Splenic anomaly	Effusion	Percentage
+	+	57
−	+	24.5
+	−	15.5
−	−	3

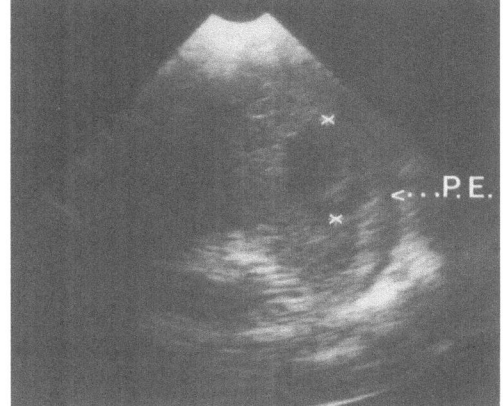

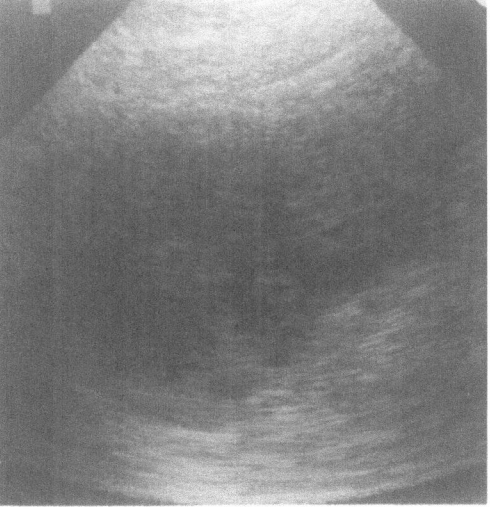

Fig. 3.5 *(above)*. Linear splenic fracture *(S; arrows)*

Fig. 3.6 *(middle)*. Blunt trauma resulted in peritoneal (41 mm between the two *crosses*) and pleural effusions *(PE)*

Fig. 3.7 *(below)*. Fractured, inhomogeneous enlarged spleen

3.2.3 Management of Splenic Trauma

Sonography of the spleen has become such a predominant imaging technique in part because it allows adoption of conservative treatment. The benefits of nonoperative management of children and adults with splenic trauma are now well recognized, both in traumatology as well as after iatrogenic injury during upper abdominal surgery.

3.2.3.1 Conservative Surgery

The adoption of protocols aimed at splenic conservation is based on several anatomic features:

- The existence of peritoneal folds allows exposure and mobilization of the spleen, splenic suture, splenorrhaphy, and elective arterial ligation.
- The vascular anatomy of the spleen, characterized by a segmental and end arterial venous system, is compatible with partial splenectomy in numerous cases; this system has been likened to a pile of plates stacked one on top of the other, with relatively few anastomoses.

The well-recognized risks of sepsis after splenectomy (Chaikof and McCabe 1985) (subphrenic abscess or pneumococcal sepsis) can be prevented by antibiotics and vaccines as well as use of such new surgical procedures as splenic hemostasis without exeresis (adhesives, powders, fibrin glue, absorbable sutures, hemostatic agents) and subtotal splenectomy.

3.2.3.2 Indications for Splenic Ultrasonography

Owing to the antixenic role of the spleen and the increasing popularity of conservative treatment, four general situations can be defined in which the role of ultrasonography depends on the clinical context:

- Large collections: surgical decisions have priority to avoid missing an associated lesion(s) requiring emergency laparotomy.
- Moderate collections with an apparently isolated splenic injury: the patient can be followed-up by both physical examinations and ultrasonography once vital signs have been stabilized.
- Solitary splenic injuries: an excellent indication for sonographic surveillance during the period of hospitalization.
- Incomplete or unsatisfactory sonographic examination: priority must be given to clinical findings during reanimation.

Ultrasonography appears particularly well suited to detection of delayed splenic rupture, which can be unpredictable: modifications in the echo patterns on serial sonograms (reflecting expansion or the formation of intraparenchymal or subcapsular hematomas, for example) can be visualized early enough for appropriate surgical intervention.

3.2.4 Patterns of Lesion Evolution

The various echo patterns demonstrated for free intraperitoneal fluid reflect the different stages of evolution of blood collections with time (Fig. 3.8). Of course, an isolated modification in a focal intrasplenic lesion is of no value in itself: most such images disappear spontaneously over a period of several weeks or months (Freeman et al. 1982). Reorganization of the splenic bed can lead to the formation of clinically asymptomatic pseudocysts: when discovered some time after more or less explicit injury, there are several differential diagnoses: traumatic splenic cyst, parasitic cyst, dystrophic cyst of doubtful pathogenesis (possibly due to an earlier injury), or underlying hematologic disorder. Sonographic information in favor of one etiology or another is extremely limited (Hertzanu and Mendelsohn 1984).

Spontaneous local complications (superinfection or organized hematoma) remain a problem, especially in patients managed nonsurgically. Splenic puncture under ultrasonic guidance has been suggested as a means of avoiding splenectomy (Epstein and Omar 1983; Lupien and Sauerbrei 1984). Formation of a purulent collection in the splenic bed is an additional risk in splenectomized patients (Delfraissy et al. 1982): this is an excellent indication for puncture, followed by evacuation, drainage, and local treatment (Fig. 3.9). Collections of sterile serous fluid are also fairly com-

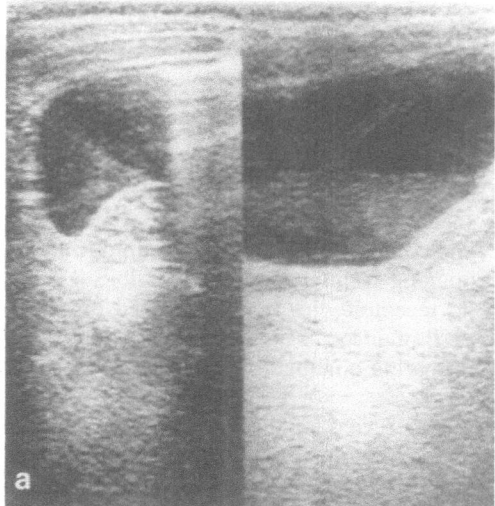

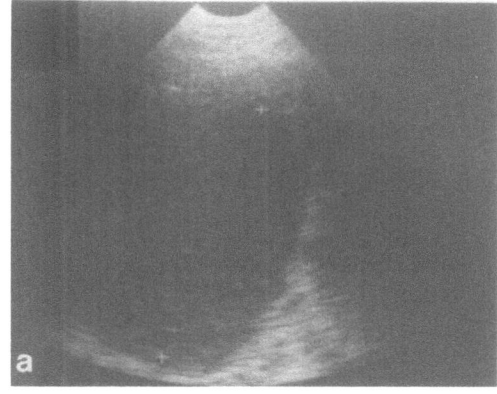

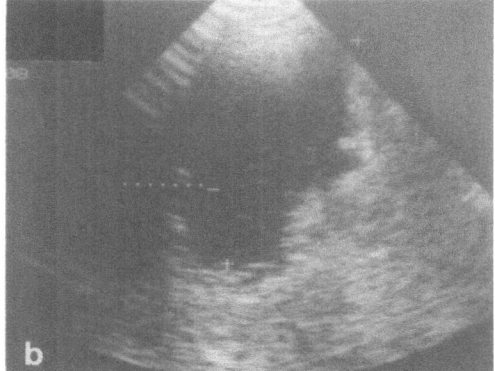

Fig. 3.9 a, b. Suppuration in a splenectomy bed: image before puncture (83 mm between the two *crosses*) (**a**) and during drainage (60 mm between the two *crosses*) (**b**)

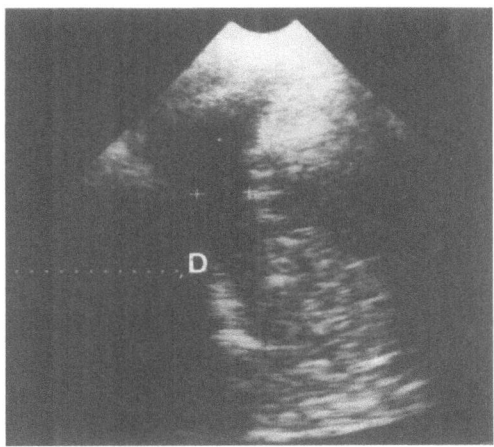

Fig. 3.8 a, b. Mixed effusion, with an air level between the fluid phase and the lower echogenic phase (clot) (**a**); focal hematoma at the lower pole of the spleen (**b**)

Fig. 3.10. Sterile postoperative collection (11 days after splenectomy). *D*, diaphragm; 17 mm between the two *crosses*

mon: these asymptomatic collections have a completely fluid echo pattern, and tend to resorb in two to three weeks (Fig.3.10).

Postoperative follow-up sonograms can be a source of modified images as well:

- Compensatory hypertrophy of an accessory spleen
- Patterns generated by certain types of sutures (hyperechoic lines) and local conservative treatments (Figs.3.11 and 3.12)

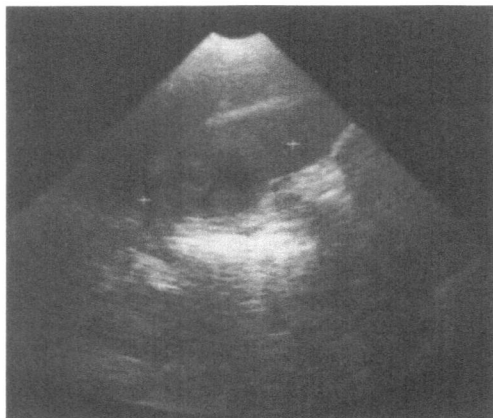

Fig.3.11. Small residual hematoma in a sutured spleen (echogenic line); 73 mm between the two *crosses*

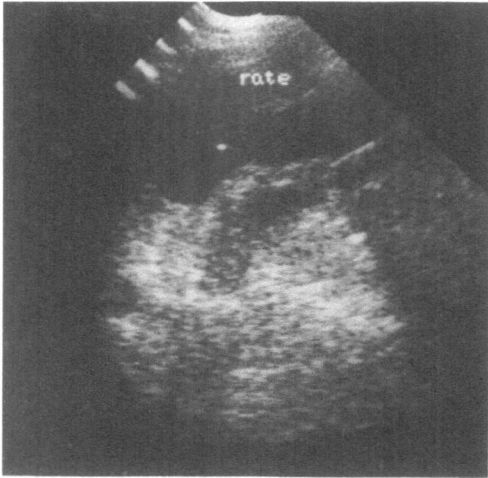

Fig.3.12. Hyperechoic appearance of a small sutured wound. *rate,* spleen

3.2.5 Reliability of Splenic Sonography and Differential Diagnosis

3.2.5.1 Value of Ultrasonography

The reliability of splenic ultrasonography cannot be defined by strict objective criteria: prospective double-blind studies for evaluation and comparison of ultrasonography with other imaging techniques are impossible. Likewise, no recent studies have compared present-day performances of ultrasound with anatomic information obtained by laparotomy in large series.

In our review of the literature, the sensitivity of splenic sonography varied with the examiner and the severity of sonographic criteria retained for diagnostic purposes. Ultrasonography is very sensitive for detection of peritoneal effusions, but is less so for actual splenic lesions. However, not all authors have included the performances of modern sector scanners in their studies (Amici et al. 1982; Bosc et al. 1984; Weill et al. 1981). Sonographer expertise can also affect the technique's sensitivity (Filiatrault et al. 1984).

Utilization of ultrasonography in an emergency situation is aimed primarily at detecting hemoperitoneum, the major indication for laparotomy. The examiner does not always have the time to localize the responsible organ. Halbfass et al. (1981), for example, reported that actual splenic lesions were diagnosed in only 50% of patients with hemoperitoneum, whereas more thorough ultrasound examination during the same period of 25 patients without hemoperitoneum diagnosed the affected organ in 22 cases.

3.2.5.2 Differential Diagnosis

False-positive errors are rare with splenic ultrasonography. However, the differential diagnosis can prove difficult in patients with non-hemorrhagic intraperitoneal fluid (ascites, urinoma) or a preexisting focal splenic lesion (infarct, inflammatory process, tumor, dystrophic pathology). Reference to the clinical context can correct the diagnosis, but several situations involve special problems:

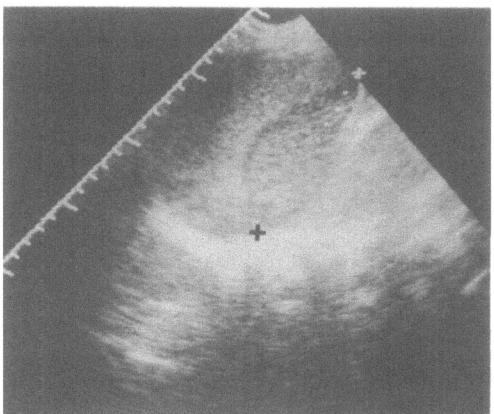

Fig. 3.13. Hilar clot caused by mesenteric rupture with hemoperitoneum (false positive); spleen unharmed (102 mm between the two *crosses*)

- A septated abscess in the process of organization will be imaged as a defect with an acoustic shadow, owing to the presence of air. In some cases, however, ultrasonically guided puncture is required for definite diagnosis (Halbfass et al. 1981): pus and/or blood may be produced, especially after delayed splenic rupture complicated by infection. Diagnosis remains problematic when an anechoic clotted hematoma fails to produce any material on puncture.
- Focal juxtasplenic effusions can be differentiated from subcapsular hematomas on the basis of image modification with shifts in the patient's position: hemoperitoneum will be displaced whereas hematomas will not. Analysis of hilar lesions is occasionally decisive: subcapsular hematomas are delimited by vascular elements whereas hemoperitoneum will completely surround the hilar vessels, creating the "drowned hilus" sign (Weill et al. 1981). Of course, this is true only if the hemoperitoneum is due to splenic rupture. As mentioned earlier, though, such sonographic patterns provide only indirect evidence of abdominal visceral injury: they are not diagnostic in themselves (Fig. 3.13).

3.3 Other Diagnostic Techniques

3.3.1 Peritoneal Lavage

Although peritoneal lavage was justified when first introduced, well before the advent of modern imaging modalities, the technique has numerous limitations:

- False-positive errors due to retroperitoneal hematoma (lavage is positive in one-third of patients with pelvic fractures) or injury during insertion of the trochar needle (Hertzanu and Mendelsohn 1984; Hicken et al. 1981)
- Negative findings in cases of nonruptured subcapsular hematoma
- A nonnegligible risk (up to 8%) of secondary complications (Halbfass et al. 1981; Hauenstein et al. 1982).

Because ultrasonography is just as sensitive as peritoneal lavage for diagnosis of hemoperitoneum, and is also atraumatic, noninvasive, and repeatable, it is generally the preferred technique. Moreover, ultrasonography can sometimes localize the source of bleeding and can evaluate the amount of hemoperitoneum.

3.3.2 Liver-Spleen Scintigraphy

Radionuclide liver and spleen scanning using technetium-labeled heated red cells is a noninvasive technique with an overall reliability of the order of 90% (Danais et al. 1984; Kaufman et al. 1984). However, this relatively economical technique has several important drawbacks:

- False-negative errors linked to the limit of detector resolution (1-2 cm)
- False-positive errors due to anatomic variants in splenic morphology (up to 7% of cases)
- Neither hemoperitoneum nor associated visceral lesions can be evaluated
- Rarely suited for use in emergency situations

By contrast, scintigraphy is indicated for the follow-up of patients managed nonsurgically, for evaluation of accessory spleens (Babcock and Kaufman 1983; Hertzanu and Mendel-

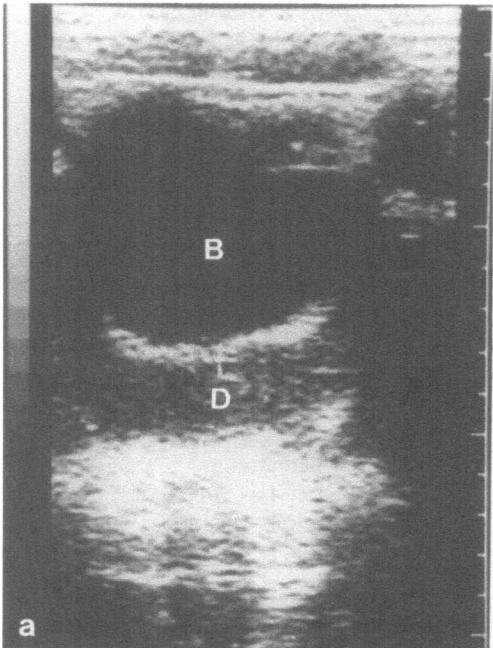

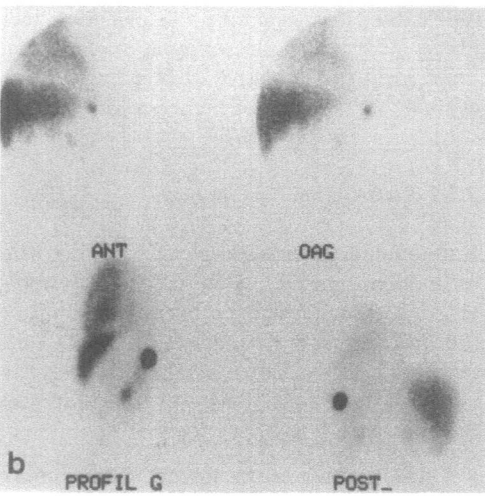

Fig. 3.14a, b. Transverse pelvic sonogram showing an echogenic effusion in the pouch of Douglas (**a**); *B*, bladder; *D*, pouch of Douglas. Poorly visible splenic contusion. An accessory spleen conserved at splenectomy shows radionuclide uptake on this follow-up scintiscan 3 months later (**b**): *ant*, anterior; *OAG*, left anterior oblique; *profil G*, left lateral; *post*, posterior

sohn 1984) and for examination of the severely injured upper left quadrant when localization of anatomic structures is particularly difficult (Fig. 3.14).

3.3.3 Computed Tomography (CT)

CT is an excellent technique for the investigation of splenic trauma as it can reliably demonstrate a wide range of lesions (Babcock and Kaufman 1983; Berger and Kuhn 1981; Jeffrey et al. 1981; Korobkin et al. 1978; Mall and Kaiser 1981; Taylor and Rosenfeld 1984):

- Direct signs of splenic fracture
- Deformation of the splenic contour by a subcapsular hematoma, which will appear hypodense in comparison to the normal parenchyma; such lesions do not enhance with contrast media (Fig. 3.15), but may become isodense during clot retraction.
- Intraperitoneal fluid: capsular rupture is always accompanied by fluid in the perisplenic region, especially at the lower pole, and almost always by fluid in Morison's pouch and the right paracolic gutter. The homogeneous density of fresh blood (45 HU) allows differentiation from ascites or a urinoma.
- Associated lesions in patients with multiple injuries (skull, thorax, abdomen) can frequently be detected during the same examination session.

CT is not hindered by bone barriers or intestinal gas, and numerous authors consider it the technique of choice for initial workups and follow-up examinations (Kaufman et al. 1984; Klels et al. 1983). However, CT can be difficult to perform for polytraumatized patients who cannot be easily moved and for individuals requiring sedation (especially children).

3.3.4 Angiography

When indicated, selective arteriography of the spleen has been considered the technique of reference for investigation of blunt splenic trauma. Certain authors (Fisher et al. 1981) have suggested a classification for splenic lesions based on angiographic patterns:

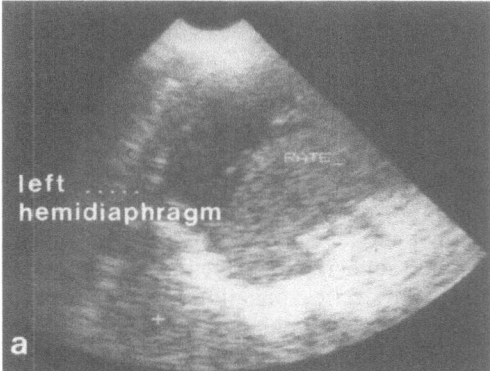

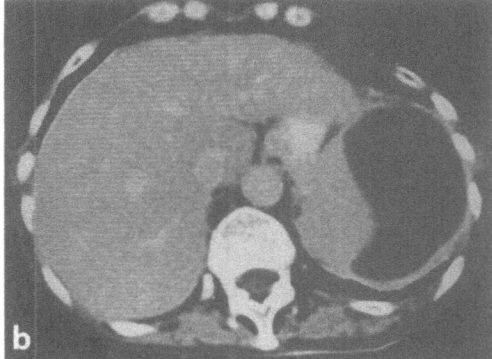

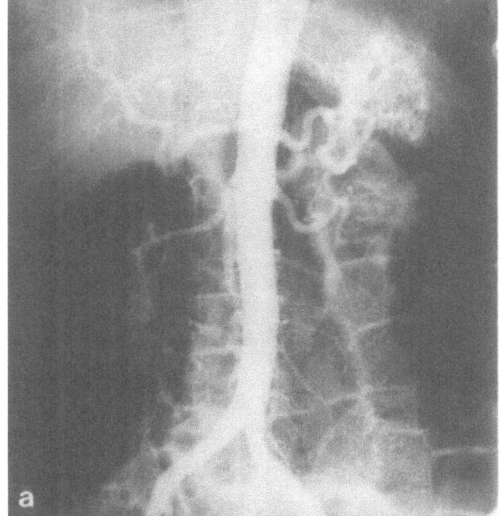

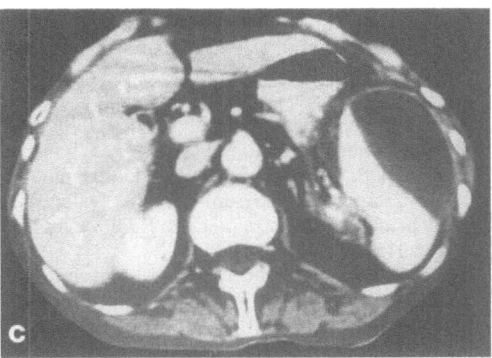

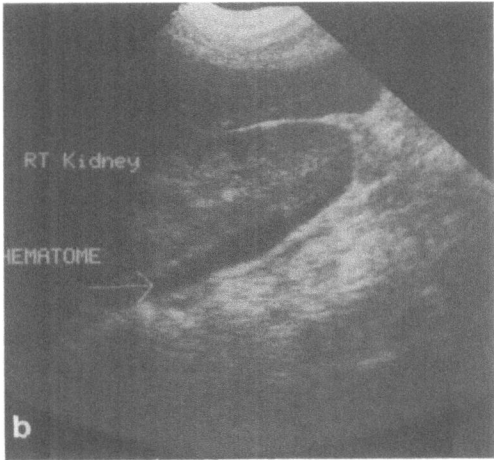

Fig. 3.15 a–c. Ultrasound (a) and CT (b, c) images of a subcapsular hematoma. *Rate,* spleen

Fig. 3.16 a, b. Arteriogram obtained for posttraumatic hematuria and subnormal intravenous pyelography. Discovery of a traumatized spleen with an extensive avascular defect due to a perisplenic hematoma (a); sonogram of a right perirenal hematoma (b)

- Severe trauma: disruption of main arterial branches, fragmented splenic parenchyma, extensive avascular defect(s)
- Intermediate trauma: intra- or extrasplenic contrast extravasation, vast avascular defect(s), subcapsular or extrasplenic hematomas
- Minor trauma: small avascular zones (less than 1 cm) or limited areas of diffuse or focal contrast extravasation

Use of such a classification may facilitate patient management. Angiography is indicated when discrepancies exist between clinical findings and other imaging studies, but the technique is both invasive and time-consuming. Moreover, angiographic findings are not always well correlated with histologic data, and the technique cannot detect hemoperitoneum outside of the splenic bed or quantify the amount of blood present. By contrast, angiog-

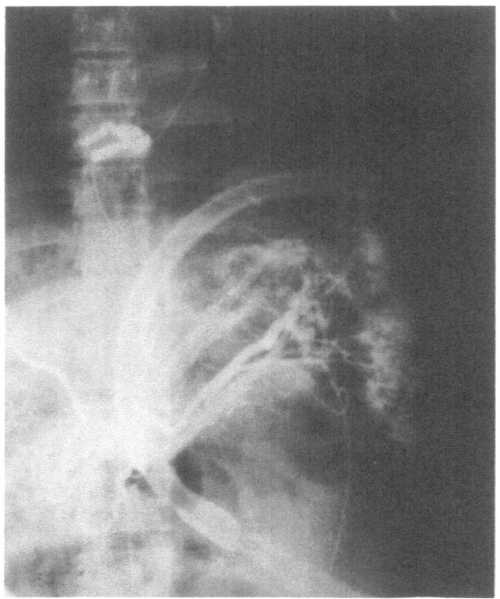

Fig. 3.17. Incidental arteriographic finding during exploration of a patient with blunt injury of the right kidney: appearance of the dislocated splenic pulp

raphy is indispensable during pretreatment workups when conservative management is being considered for patients with a splenic lesion or an associated soft tissue injury (Figs. 3.16 and 3.17). Angiography is also necessary before interventional arteriography, namely of the liver or kidneys.

3.4 Conclusion

Overall, the limitations of sonographic examination of splenic trauma are those of the technique in general:

- Possibility that the ultrasound study is not adequate
- Possibility of discrepancies between the clinical course and biological findings (rare instances of false-negative and false-positive errors with ultrasonography)

Despite these limitations, ultrasonography has unquestionable advantages:

- Nearly 100% sensitivity for detection of free intraperitoneal fluid, even for very small collections

- Reliable diagnosis of a high percentage of splenic lesions
- Best technique for surveillance of patients treated nonsurgically and patients who do not undergo surgery immediately

A certain degree of uncertainty still persists, however, when trying to fit splenic ultrasonography into a clinical management protocol: Should sonography be the first technique used after physical examination of the patient and stabilization of vital signs? Should it be performed before CT, or has it been completely supplanted by CT? There are no universal solutions, because the strategy adopted at each trauma center will depend on such parameters as patient recruitment, available equipment, personnel qualification, and existing work routines.

3.5 References

Amici F, Busilacchi P, De Nigris E, Giuseppetti GM, Legeza G, Stramentinoli A, Testasecca D (1982) Closed abdominal injuries: the diagnostic reliability of ultrasonics. Radiol Med 68: 5–10

Aufschnaiter M, Kofler H (1983) Sonographische Akutdiagnostik beim Polytrauma. Akt Traumatol 13: 55–57

Asher WM, Parvin S, Virgilio RW, Haber K (1976) Echographic evaluation of splenic injury after blunt trauma. Radiology 118: 411–415

Babcock DS, Kaufman RA (1983) Ultrasonography and computed tomography in the evaluation of the acutely ill pediatric patient. Radiol Clin North AM 21: 527–550

Berger PE, Kuhn JP (1981) CT of blunt abdominal trauma in childhood. AJR 136: 105–110

Bosc O, Bensoussan AL, Morin JF, Blanchard H, Filiatrault D, Danais S (1984) Traumatismes spléniques: orientation thérapeutique à propos de 46 cas. Chir Pédiatr 25: 1–5

Chaikof EL, Mc Cabe CJ (1985) Fatal overwhelming postsplenectomy infection. Am J Surg 149: 534–539

Danais S, Dumont M, Taillefer R, Soucy JP, Morin JF, Bensoussan A, Filiatrault D (1984) Les lésions spléniques traumatiques: rôle de la scintigraphie et traitement non opératoire. Union Méd Can 113: 57–64

Delfraissy JF, Brivet F, Dormont J (1982) Complications infectieuses et splénectomies. Chirurgie 108: 327–331

Epstein BM, Omar GM (1983) Infective complications of splenic trauma. Clin Radiol 34: 91–94

Farthmann EH, Harder F, Dürig M, Schwemmle K, Seufert RM, Encke A, Siewert JR (1985) Betrachten Sie die Replantation von Milzgewebe nach Splenektomie wegen traumatischer Milzruptur bereits als Routine? Langencks Arch Chir 365: 147-152

Federle MP, Jeffrey RB (1983) Hemoperitoneum studied by computed tomography. Radiology 148: 137-192

Filiatrault D, Graignon A, Boisvert J, Morin JF, Bensoussan A, Soucy JP, Danais S (1984) Le rôle de l'échographie dans le traumatisme splénique chez l'enfant. J Radiol 65: 79-83

Fisher RG, Foucar K, Estrada R, Ben Menachem Y (1981) Splenic rupture in blunt trauma. Radiol Clin North Am 19: 141-165

Freeman LD, Anderson DS, Greaney RB, Kilcheski TS, McAdams SA (1982) Non-operative management of delayed splenic rupture in an adult. Dig Dis Sci 27: 171-174

Halbfass HJ, Wimmer B, Hauenstein KH, Zavisic D (1981) Ultraschall - Diagnostik des stumpfen Bauchtraumas. Fortschr Med 99: 1681-1685

Hauenstein KH, Wimmer B, Billmann P, Noldge G, Zavisic D (1982) Die Rolle der Sonographie beim stumpfen Bauchtrauma. Radiologe 22: 106-111

Hertzanu Y, Mendelsohn DB (1984) Delayed splenic rupture: a true entity. Clin Radiol 35: 393-396

Hicken P, Sauerbrei EE, Cooperberg PL (1981) Ultrasonic coronal scanning of left upper quadrant. J Can Assoc Radiol 32: 107-110

Jeffrey RB, Laing FC, Federle MP, Goodman PC (1981) Computed tomography of splenic trauma. Radiology 141: 729-732

Johnson MA, Cooperberg PL, Boisvert J, Stoller JL, Winrob H (1981) Spontaneous splenic rupture in infectious mononucleosis: sonographic diagnosis and follow-up. AJR 136: 111-114

Jones TK, Walsh JW, Maull KI (1983) Diagnostic imaging in blunt trauma of the abdomen. Surg Gynecol Obstet 157: 389-398

Kaufman RA, Towbin R, Babcock DS, Gelfand MJ, Guice KS, Oldham KT, Noseworthy J (1984) Upper abdominal trauma in children: imaging evaluation. AJR 142: 449-460

Klels E, Pringot J, Dardenne AN, Dautrebande J, Coppens JP (1983) Computed tomography in abdominal and thoracic trauma - comparison with abdominal ultrasonography and chest radiography. J Belge Radiol 66: 31-38

Korobkin M, Moss AA, Callen PW, Demartini WS, Kaiser JA (1978) Computed tomography of subcapsular splenic hematoma. Radiology 129: 441-445

Kuhn FP, Schreyer T, Schild H, Klose K, Gunther R (1983) Sonographie beim stumpfen Bauchtrauma. Fortsch Röntgenstr 139: 310-313

Lupien C, Sauerbrei EE (1984) Healing in the traumatized spleen: sonographic investigation. Radiology 151: 181-185

Mall JC, Kaiser JA (1980) CT diagnosis of splenic laceration. AJR 134: 265-269

Schulz RD, Willi U (1983) Ultraschalldiagnostik nach stumpfen Bauchverletzungen im Kindesalter. Ultraschall 4: 154-159

Solheim K, Hoivik B (1985) Changing trends in the diagnosis and management of rupture of the spleen. Injury 16: 221-226

Taylor CR, Rosenfield AT (1984) Limitations of computed tomography in the recognition of delayed splenic rupture. J Comput Assist Tomog 8: 1205-1207

van Sonnenberg E, Simeone JF, Mueller PR, Wittenberg J, Hall DA, Ferrucci JT (1983) Sonographic appearance of hematoma in liver, spleen and kidney: a clinical, pathologic and animal study. Radiology 147: 507-510

Verge-Garret J, Ptak Y, Wertel F, Lafaye C, Vanneuville G, Richard Y, Ronayette H (1983) Apport de l'échographie dans le diagnostic et la surveillance des lésions traumatiques hépato-spléniques de l'enfant. JEMU 4: 23-28

Viscomi GN, Gonzalez R, Taylor JW, Grade M (1980) Ultrasonic evaluation of hepatic and splenic trauma. Arch Surg 115: 320-321

Weill F, Bihr E, Rohmer P, Zeltner F, Lemouel A, Perriguey G (1981) Ultrasonic study of hepatic and splenic traumatic lesions. Eur J Radiol 1: 245-249

Wilson RL, Rogers WF, Shaub MS, Birnbaum W (1978) Splenic subcapsular hematoma - ultrasonic diagnosis. West J Med 128: 6-8

4 Splenic Tumors

J. N. Bruneton, C. Balu-Maestro, J. Drouillard, F. Normand, J. G. Fuzibet

Tumors of the spleen are uncommon and often asymptomatic. Most malignant splenic tumors have a lymphomatous etiology. The main risk with benign lesions is hemorrhage. Although the sonographic features of splenic tumors are usually nonspecific, the sensitivity of the technique appears satisfactory, except for lymphomas. Ultrasound detection of focal nonlymphomatous lesions warrants further investigation by computed tomography for accurate diagnosis.

4.1 Malignant Tumors

Splenic malignancies caused by direct extension of a neoplastic process in a contiguous structure have been excluded from this review. Lymphomas account for the majority of primary malignant splenic tumors. Meyer et al. (1983) cited the Bostick study (1945) of 17707 autopsies and 68820 splenectomies which found only 5 primary splenic tumors (including 2 malignant non-Hodgkin lymphomas) and the 14-year-study by Das Gupta which mentioned only 10 primary splenic malignancies (9 non-Hodgkin lymphomas, 1 angiosarcoma).

4.1.1 Lymphomas (Figs. 4.1 to 4.12)

Primary non-Hodgkin lymphoma (NHL) and Hodgkin's disease (HD) of the spleen represent less than 1% of all lymphomatous disease sites. NHL clearly predominates (approximately 75% of all primary splenic lymphomas; Bruneton et al. 1986). One-third of all lymphoma patients develop secondary splenic involvement at some point in their disease course; 90% of secondary splenic lesions are of an infiltrative nature, and thus hard to diag-

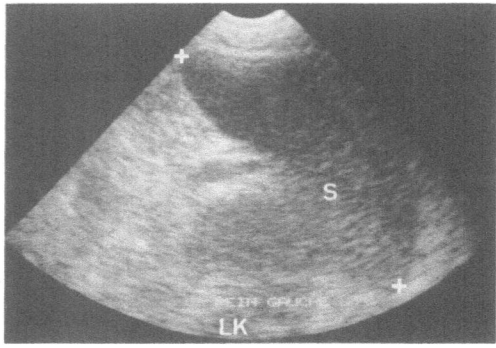

Fig. 4.1. Non-Hodgkin lymphoma (NHL); homogeneous splenomegaly (transverse scan). *LK (rein gauche),* left kidney

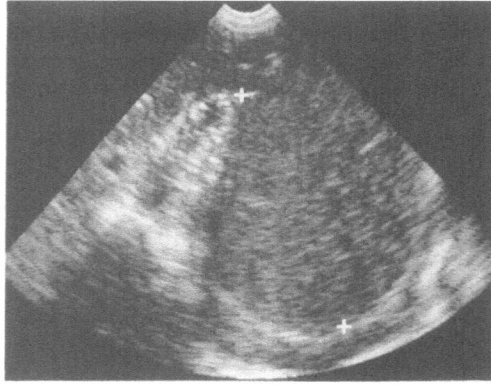

Fig. 4.2. Hodgkin's disease (HD); homogeneous splenomegaly (transverse scan)

nose (Balu et al. 1984; Bruneton et al. 1986). Splenomegaly, an inconstant and nonspecific feature of splenic malignancies, can result in a 10- to 20-fold increase in the weight of the normal spleen (Bruneton et al. 1983).

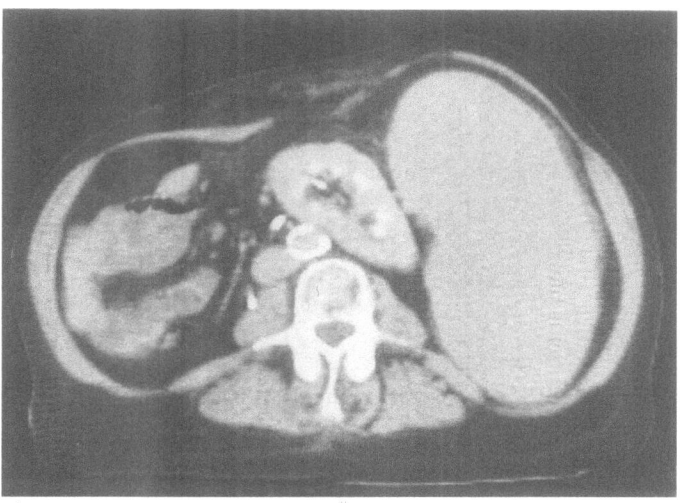

Fig. 4.3. NHL: homogeneous splenomegaly with medial displacement of the left kidney (CT scan)

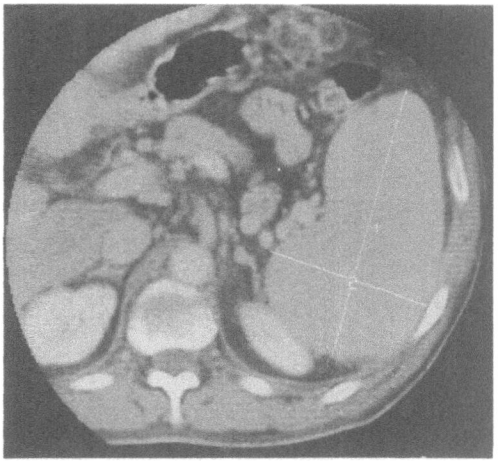

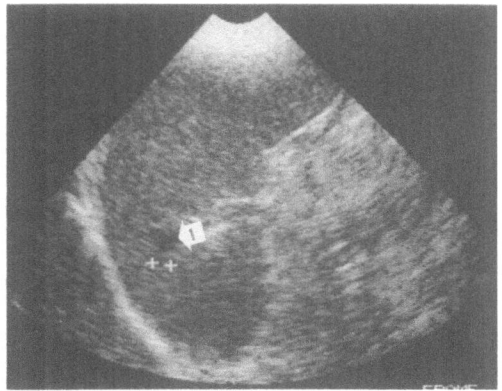

Fig. 4.4 NHL: homogeneous splenomegaly (88 mm × 150 mm)

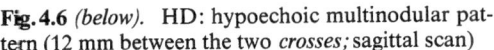

Fig. 4.5 *(above).* NHL: small hypoechoic splenic nodule (*arrow:* 7 mm between the two adjacent *crosses;* sagittal scan)

Fig. 4.6 *(below).* HD: hypoechoic multinodular pattern (12 mm between the two *crosses;* sagittal scan)

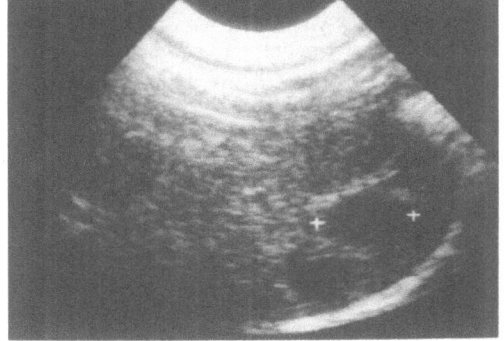

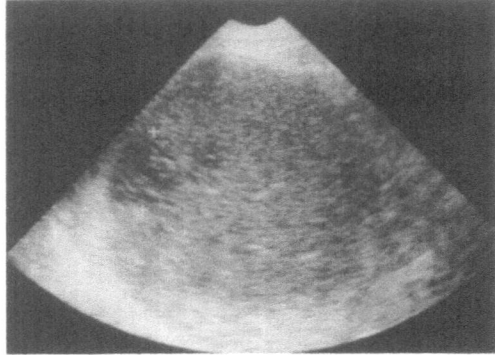

Fig. 4.7. NHL: multinodular pattern (31 mm between the two *crosses;* sagitt* scan)

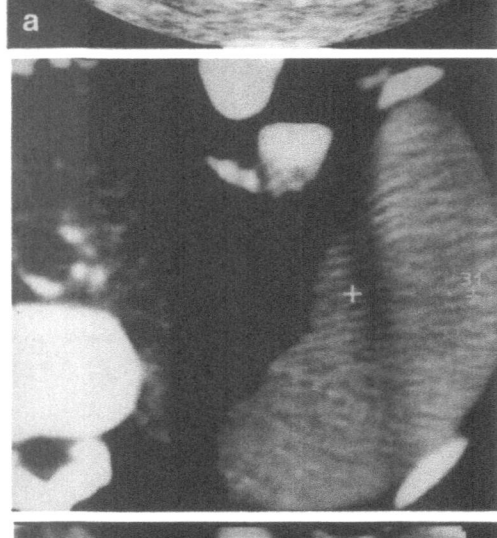

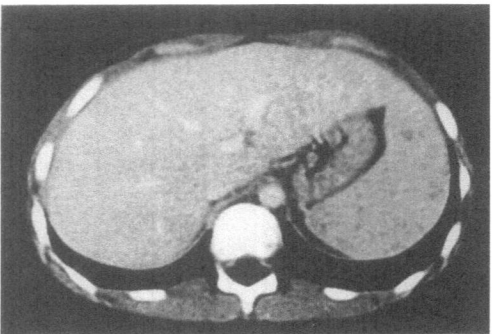

Fig. 4.8. HD: micronodular pattern (less than 1 cm diameter)

Fig. 4.9. See p. 49

Fig. 4.9. See p. 49

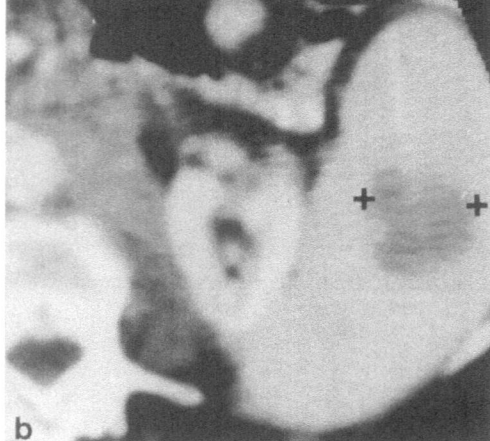

Fig. 4.10 a, b. Waldenström's disease: two hyperechoic splenic nodules (3 cm between the two *crosses*) on a sagittal sonogram; on CT (pre- and postcontrast images) – the larger lesion is hypodense

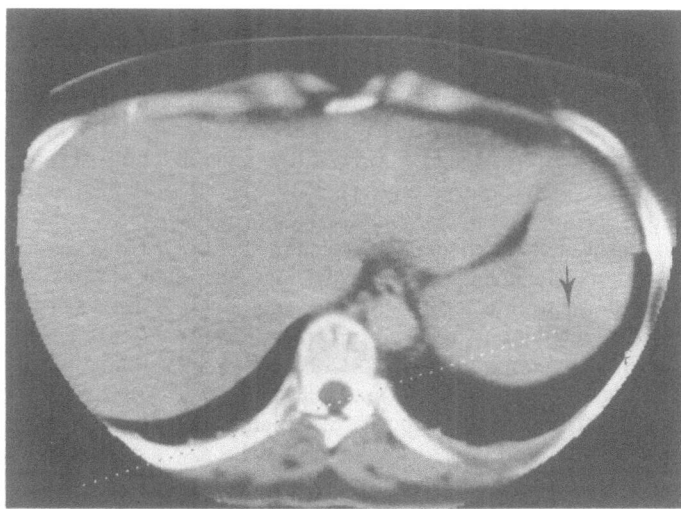

Fig. 4.9. NHL: 3 cm diameter hypodense splenic nodule *(arrow)*; the spleen was normal in size

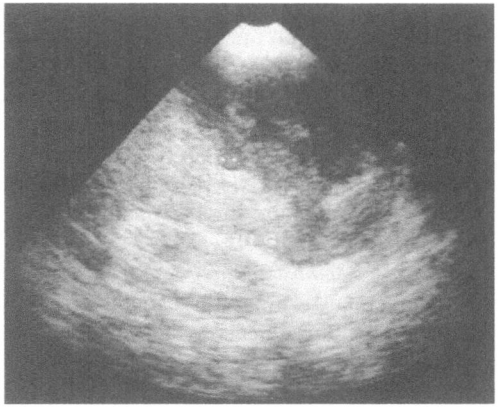

Fig. 4.11. NHL: splenomegaly with a hypoechoic heterogeneous pattern (sagittal scan): this patient presented with left upper quadrant pain; at autopsy, the lower part of the spleen showed infarction

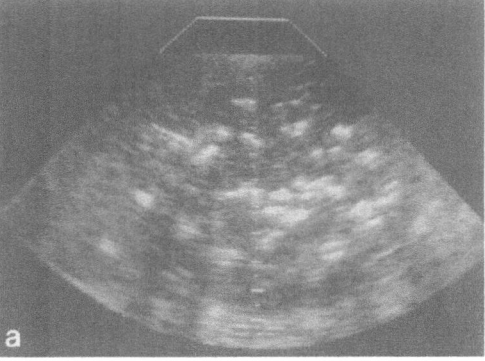

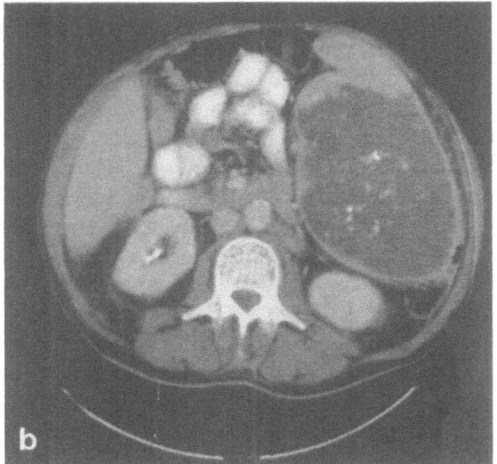

Fig. 4.12 a, b. US (**a**) and CT (**b**) study of a large old calcified and homogeneous infarction of part of the spleen

4.1.1.1 Non-Hodgkin Lymphoma

Thirty-two percent of NHL patients have splenic involvement at initial presentation. The incidence is particularly high (64%) in patients with nodular, poorly differentiated lymphocytic disease (Thomas et al. 1982).

The spleen generally has a normal sonographic appearance. Homogeneous splenomegaly is common. The splenic parenchyma may be either more or less echogenic than the liver: contact scanning is required for precise evaluation (Bruneton et al. 1983). Comparison of the organ's dimension on serial sonograms allows retrospective diagnosis of splenic involvement. Response to treatment can be assessed in the same manner. In a limited percentage of cases, visualization of single or multiple focal lesions that are less echoic than the normal splenic parenchyma readily suggests NHL. Solitary complex hypoechoic defects indicate recent infarction, whereas more or less extensive hyperechoic lesions correspond to long-standing infarcts. Individuals with a coagulopathy may present an anechoic peripheral lesion representing a subcapsular hematoma. In rare instances, a large complex mass with smooth margins may be visible. Adenopathies at the splenic hilus are often associated with splenic lesions (Bruneton et al. 1986; De Graaff et al. 1979; Mittelstaedt and Partain 1980; Solbiati et al. 1983). The sensitivity of ultrasonography for the detection of splenic NHL is relatively satisfactory: 77.8% (De Graaff et al. 1979; Glees et al. 1977).

Computed tomography may fail to recognize splenic NHL; a normal CT scan thus does not rule out the possibility of involvement. CT will usually demonstrate homogeneous splenomegaly. On rare occasions, small (2–3 cm) lesions of lower density than the normal splenic parenchyma are visualized. A single large mass of decreased CT attenuation is another possibility (Anjou et al. 1983; Federle and Moss 1983; Meyer et al. 1983; Piekarski et al. 1980). While CT can easily evaluate splenic size, the normal dimensions of the organ vary so greatly from one individual to the next that size is difficult to retain as a diagnostic criterion (Federle and Moss 1983). Furthermore, one-third of patients with splenic NHL have a normal-sized spleen. The threshold for detection of lymphomatous nodules is 0.5–1 cm, with or without contrast material infusion (Federle and Moss 1983; Lorenz et al. 1983; Piekarski et al. 1980; Zornoza and Ginaldi 1981). Overall, CT appears of limited value for investigation of splenic NHL: estimates of the technique's sensitivity range from 17%–25% (Vermess et al. 1982; Zornoza and Ginaldi 1981). However, CT results are reportedly improved by intravenous injection of Ethiodol (Ethiodized Oil Emulsion 13), offering a 92% detection rate for lymphomatous nodules larger than 5 mm (Thomas et al. 1982; Vermess et al. 1981, 1982). Ethiodol studies also allow detection of accessory spleens.

4.1.1.2 Hodgkin's Disease

Splenic involvement by HD is found at initial staging in 34%–42% of patients; the incidence rises to 75% in autopsy series (Sekiya et al. 1982; Thomas et al. 1982). There is no reliable correlation between splenic HD and organ size. The rate of preoperative diagnostic error varies from 30%–33% (Sekiya et al. 1982). Solitary splenic involvement by HD does not modify the outcome for a patient with a supradiaphragmatic lesion. By contrast, diagnosis of splenic lesions in NHL patients corresponds to subdiaphragmatic involvement and thus stage III disease.

Liver/spleen scintiscans can demonstrate splenic enlargement (either homogeneous or with associated filling defects). Radionuclide scanning has a predictive value of 43% for diagnosis of splenic involvement in HD (De Graaff et al. 1979). *Sonograms* are often normal. Homogeneous splenomegaly is common. Splenic HD may also be visualized as hypoechoic, frequently multiple focal lesions (Bruneton et al. 1986; De Graaff et al. 1979; Mittelstaedt and Partain 1980; Sekiya et al. 1982). After chemotherapy, the spleen may contain hyperechoic nodular defects corresponding to fibrotic areas secondary to treatment (Sekiya et al. 1982). *CT* features are nonspecific and identical to those for splenic NHL.

Despite its limitations, ultrasonography is a useful technique for the initial staging and follow-up of patients with lymphoma, and in particular those with splenic involvement.

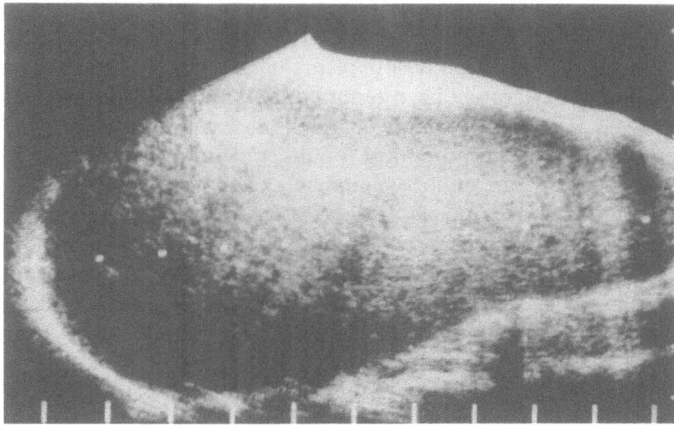

Fig. 4.13. Leukemia: homogeneous splenomegaly; sagittal diameter 32.4 cm. The entire lesion was accurately visualized and measured by contact scanning

4.1.2 Leukoses (Fig. 4.13)

Physical examination will disclose splenomegaly of variable degree. *Sonographic determination* of spleen size in patients with splenomegaly is easier with a contact scanner than with a real-time instrument.

In patients with acute leukoses, the spleen is imaged as a homogeneous, normal-sized or enlarged structure of variable echogenicity. Sonographic examination of individuals with chronic disease can reveal altered splenic architecture (Mittelstaedt and Partain 1980; Siler et al. 1980).

4.1.3 Sarcomas (Fig. 4.14)

4.1.3.1 Hemangiosarcomas

Splenic hemangiosarcoma is extremely rare. In the Das Gupta series cited by Meyer et al. (1983), only 10 primary splenic tumors were seen in a 14-year-period, and only one of these was an angiosarcoma. This type of tumor may occur either de novo, or as a primary or secondary splenic site of systemic hemangiosarcomatosis (Rappaport 1966). The frequency of simultaneous liver involvement explains the severe nature of these lesions. The natural course includes metastatic dissemination and systemic hemangiosarcomatosis; there is also

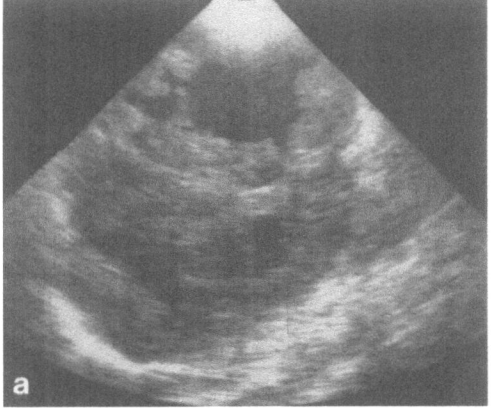

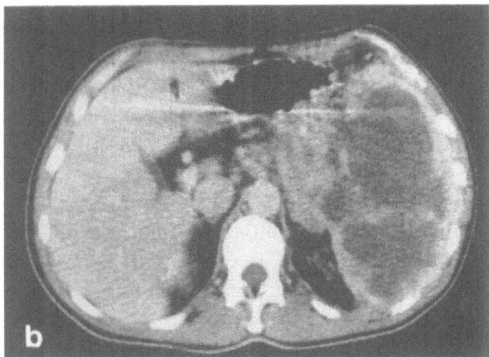

Fig. 4.14a, b. Histiocytopheosarcoma: US (**a**) and CT (**b**) study showing involvement of the entire spleen by a multinodular, necrotic pattern

a risk of intraperitoneal rupture (Rappaport 1966).

The *sonographic features* of splenic hemangiosarcoma have rarely been reported. Solbiati et al. (1983) described a large complex mass with numerous hyperechoic focal lesions, a pattern identical to that of hemangiomas except for the absence of hypoechoic zones. In the case reported by Nahman and Cunningham (1985), sonography demonstrated a huge tumor containing poorly reflective nodules, a pattern also seen with lymphoma.

Arteriograms will show multiple intratumoral vascular lakes; there are no evident tumoral vessels or tumor opacification (Kishikawa et al. 1978).

4.1.3.2 Other Sarcomas

Rhabdomyosarcoma of the spleen is exceedingly rare. In one published report (Anjou et al. 1983), clinical manifestations included long-standing fever; *CT* demonstrated an inhomogeneous lesion of the splenic bed containing both a fluid density component and dense enhancing zones. Histologic diagnosis of splenic fibrosarcoma is difficult; the differential diagnosis is angiosarcoma (Rappaport 1966).

4.1.4 Secondary Malignant Tumors
(Figs. 4.15 to 4.24)

The spleen is the site of only 2%–4% of all metastases, yet such lesions are not really rare: around 50% of all disseminated thoracic and abdominal cancers involve metastasis to the spleen (Mittelstaedt and Partain 1980; Rappaport 1966). Gross splenic metastases are seen in 67% of autopsies (Federle and Moss 1983; Piekarski et al. 1980). The major primary lesions, in order of decreasing frequency, are cancers of the lung, breast, prostate, colon and stomach, and choriocarcinoma. Approximately 50% of melanomas also metastasize to the spleen (Mittelstaedt and Partain 1980). Splenic metastases are often asymptomatic; even acute complications rarely lead to correct diagnosis. Histologic classifications distinguish between solitary (31.5%) or multiple (60%) nodular le-

sions and diffuse infiltrating lesions (8.5%; Rappaport 1966).

Ultrasonography has a high false-negative rate, probably because examination of patients with recognized cancer is oriented towards detection of hepatic and retroperitoneal metastases, and the liver is not involved in 70% of patients with splenic metastasis. Ultrasound examination of the spleen itself is thus indispensable during cancer workups. Splenic metastases usually appear hypoechoic in comparison to the normal splenic parenchyma, but

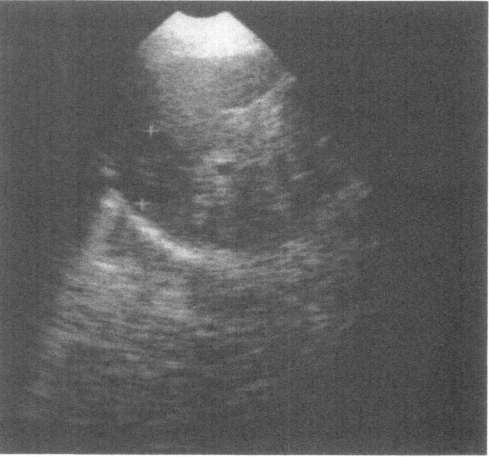

Fig. 4.15. Bronchogenic carcinoma: hypoechoic splenic metastasis (34 mm between the two *crosses*)

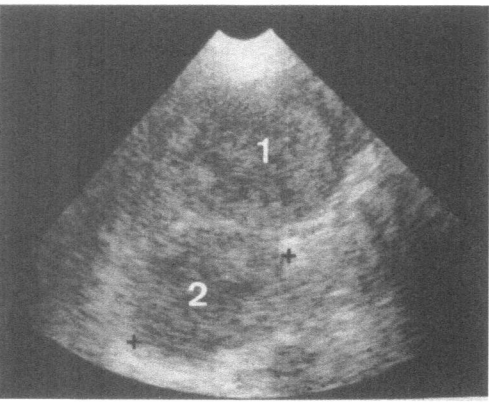

Fig. 4.16. Anaplastic bronchogenic carcinoma: splenic metastasis *(1)* and left suprarenal metastasis *(2;* 7 cm between the two *crosses;* sagittal scan)

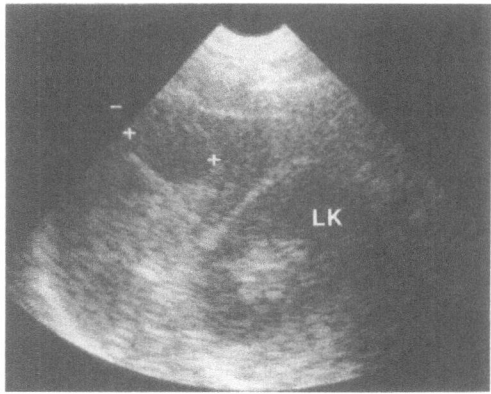

Fig. 4.17. Ovarian carcinoma: hypoechoic splenic metastasis (28 mm between the two *crosses;* sagittal scan; *LK*, left kidney)

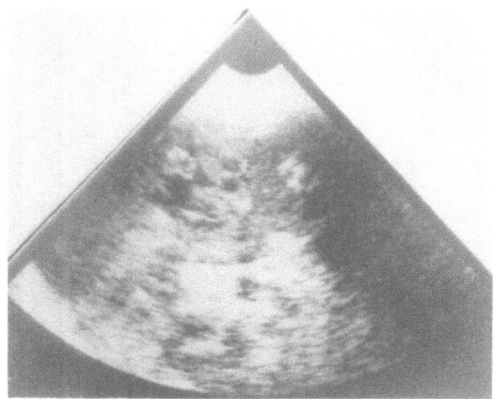

Fig. 4.19. Peritoneal myxoma: splenic metastasis (sagittal scan)

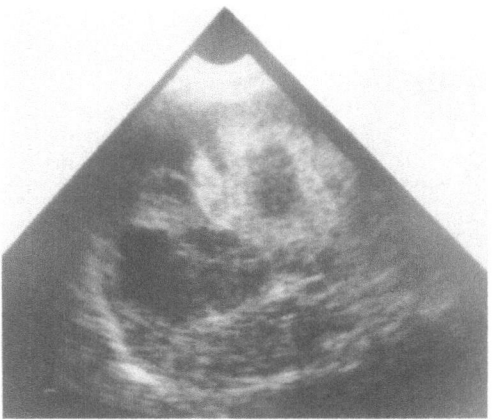

Fig. 4.18. Pheochromocytoma: large splenic metastasis with necrotic areas (sagittal scan)

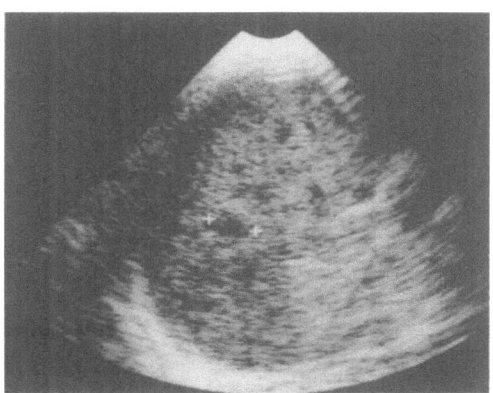

Fig. 4.20. Malignant melanoma: multinodular splenic metastases (18 mm between the two *crosses;* sagittal scan)

Fig. 4.21. Colonic carcinoma: small hyperechoic splenic metastasis (18 mm between the two *crosses;* sagittal scan)

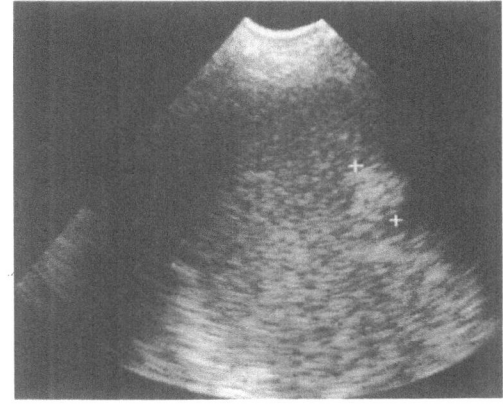

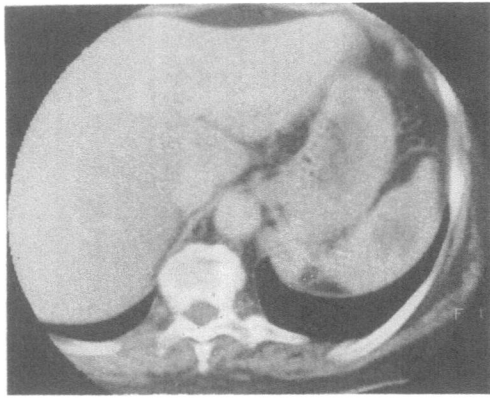

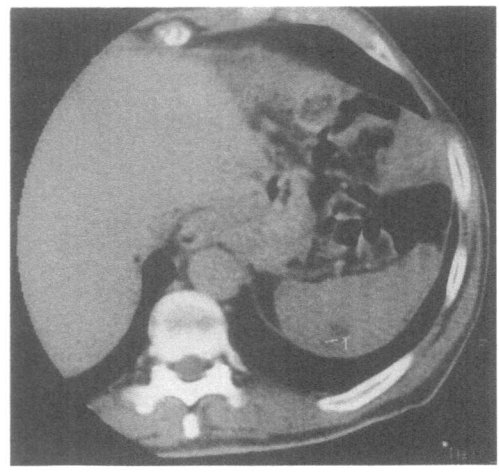

Fig. 4.22. Anaplastic bronchogenic carcinoma: hypodense splenic metastasis

Fig. 4.24. Ovarian carcinoma: small (13 mm) hypodense metastasis diagnosed by CT, confirmed by splenectomy, but undetected by ultrasonography

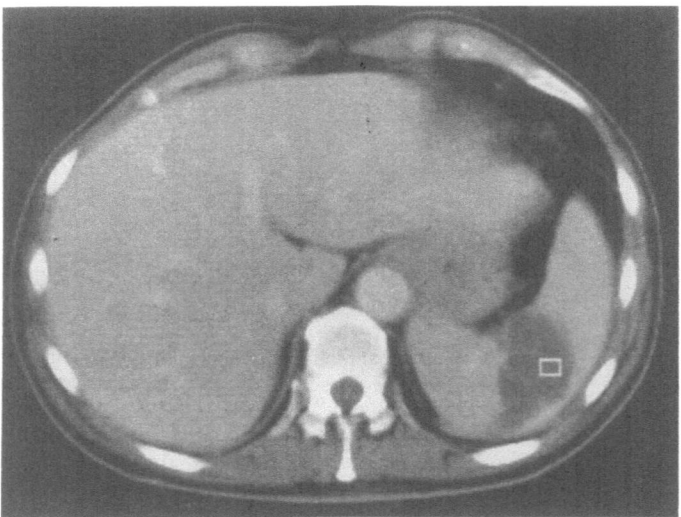

Fig. 4.23. Colonic carcinoma: hypodense splenic metastasis

less so than lymphomatous lesions. Several rare reports have described splenic metastases of ovarian and pancreatic cancer as hyperechoic and bull's-eye lesions (Bruneton et al. 1984; Mittelstaedt and Partain 1980; Murphy and Bernardino 1979; Siler et al. 1980).
Computed tomography generally demonstrates splenic metastases as rounded, nonfluid defects of decreased attenuation that do not enhance or enhance only slightly. Twenty percent of splenic metastases have an attenuation value close to 0 HU, and in 20% of cases these lesions can only be seen after intravenous injection of contrast material (Anjou et al. 1983; Bisker and McCarthy 1983; Federle and Moss 1983; Newmark 1982; Piekarski et al. 1980).

The nature of the primary tumor conditions the *arteriographic features* of splenic metastases: metastases of melanoma and uterine and bladder cancer are avascular, whereas lesions caused by renal tumors and chorioepitheliomas are vascularized (Kishikawa et al. 1978).

4.2 Benign Tumors

4.2.1 Cysts

Nonparasitic splenic cysts are rare, because over 60% of all true cysts are parasitic (hydatid cysts, the differential diagnosis for benign splenic tumors, are discussed in Chapter 6). Nonparasitic cysts undergo calcification is 11% of cases, and less than 1% involve a risk of malignant transformation (Combe et al. 1980; Issa et al. 1984). Cystic splenic lesions other than parasitic cysts can be classified as follows (Rappaport 1966):

- True (primary) cysts with a true cellular lining (epithelial, epidermoid, and dermoid cysts; endothelial and mesothelial cysts)
- False (secondary) cysts without a true cellular lining
- Enteroid cysts (a recently defined entity, Issa et al. 1984)

4.2.1.1 Epithelial Cysts (Figs. 4.25 to 4.28)

Epidermoid cysts are the most prevalent type, representing 10% of all nonparasitic true splenic cysts (Carpenter et al. 1986; Tran-Minh et al. 1980). Epithelial cysts occur primarily in children and young adults; mean age at diagnosis is 15 years. These lesions are often clinically latent; presenting symptoms may include a mass in the left upper quadrant or left upper quadrant pain radiating to the left shoulder. A large mass may compress contiguous organs. Potential complications of epithelial splenic cysts include intracystic hemorrhage (with rapid increase in spleen size and pain), intraperitoneal or intrathoracic rupture, and superinfection (Dawes and Malangoni 1986). Natural progression toward splenic enlargement and the unknown risks of malignant transformation (Issa et al. 1984) justify cura-

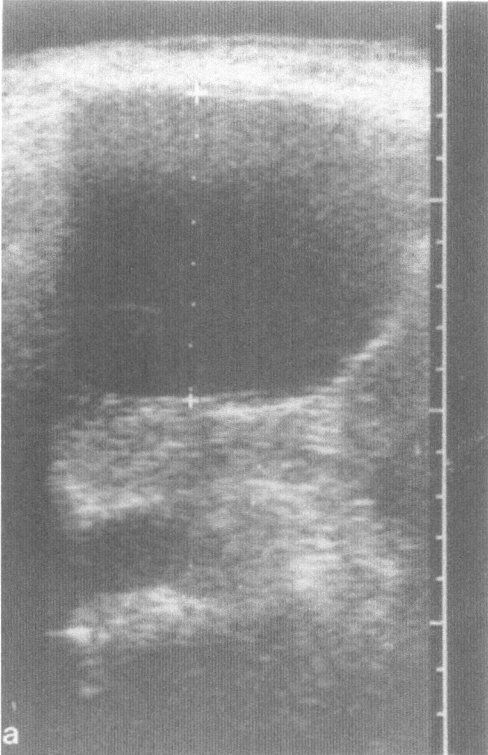

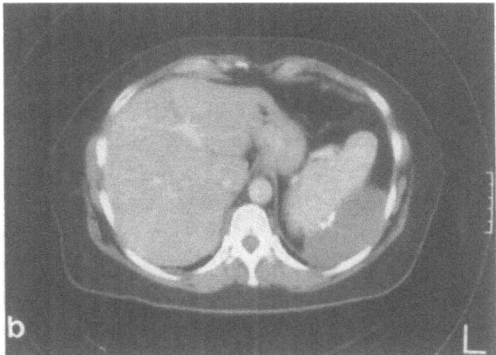

Fig. 4.25 a, b. Epithelial cyst: US (**a**) and CT (**b**) study

tive splenectomy, even though preoperative aspiration biopsy can make the diagnosis (Goldfinger et al. 1986).

Plain abdominal radiographs reveal thick, uniform intratumoral calcifications in 10% of cases (Arnold et al. 1982; Labbe et al. 1981).
Radionuclide scans can demonstrate an intrasplenic filling defect which may displace the

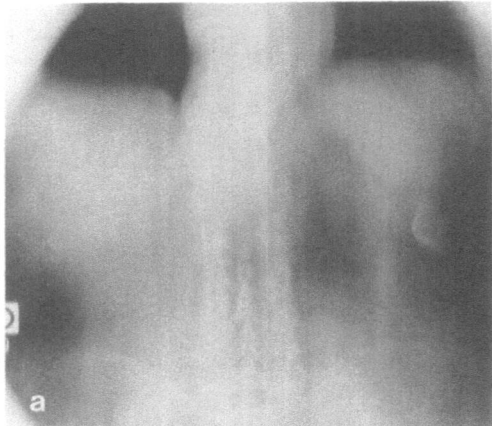

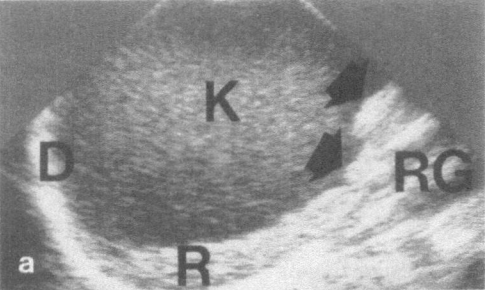

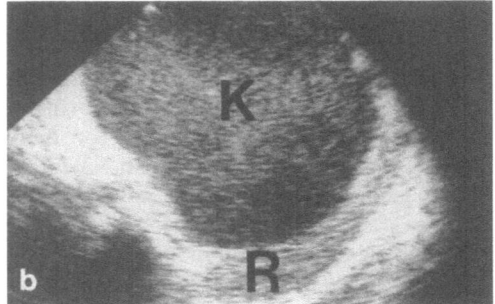

Fig. 4.28 a, b. Epidermoid cyst (**a** sagittal scan; **b** transverse scan) hypoechoic homogeneous pattern with displacement *(arrows)* of the normal spleen (*K*, cyst; *R*, spleen; *D*, diaphragm; *RG*, left kidney). (Courtesy of Dr. Tran-Minh)

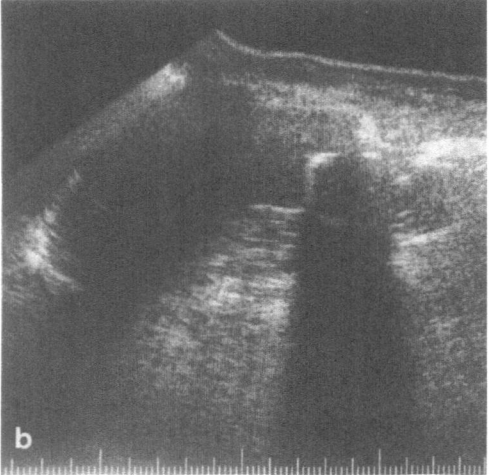

Fig. 4.26 a, b. Calcified cyst: plain film (**a**) and sonogram (**b**). (Courtesy of Dr. Matter)

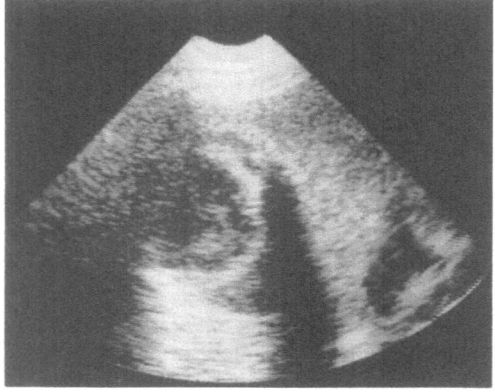

Fig. 4.27. Epidermoid cyst: partial fluid pattern with calcification (sagittal scan)

kidney. *Arteriograms* demonstrate a benign avascular process.

Sonographic features include a transsonic mass with peripheral trabeculae (Quilichini et al. 1983). Internal echoes produced by intracystic blood clots or desquamated keratine can create problems for differential diagnosis from posttraumatic and parasitic cysts (Arnold et al. 1982; Buff and Forster 1980; Solbiati et al. 1983). The typical *CT* appearance is a rounded, water density mass with sharp margins; these nonenhancing lesions occasionally contain septations (Anjou et al. 1983; Arnold et al. 1982; Garcia Correa et al. 1985; Piekarski et al. 1980).

4.2.1.2 Endothelial Cysts (Figs. 4.29 and 4.30)

These congenital lesions, which include both simple serous cysts and polycystic disease, account for approximately 10% of all nonparasitic true cysts (Rappaport 1966). Asymptomatic splenomegaly is the most common phys-

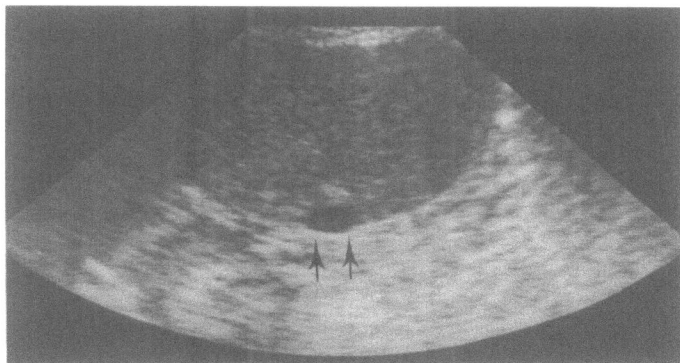

Fig. 4.29. Serous cyst: small anechoic pattern (*arrows;* sagittal scan)

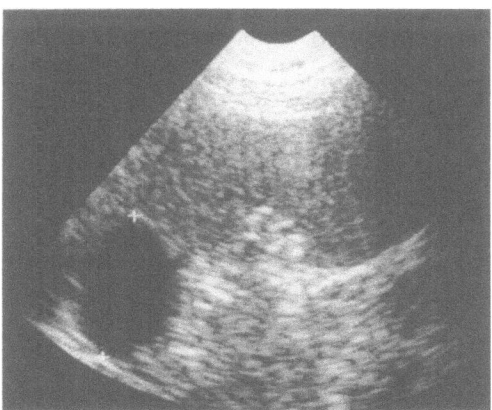

Fig. 4.30. Serous cyst: anechoic rounded lesion (38 mm between the two *crosses;* sagittal scan)

ical finding; pain or a tumoral syndrome occurs on rare occasions. Endothelial cysts run a benign course. Certain authors have advocated evacuation by ultrasound-guided puncture (Solbiati et al. 1983), but this technique remains controversial owing to the risk of hemorrhage (Quilichini et al. 1983).

Sonographically, endothelial cysts present as single or multiple transsonic masses, occasionally associated with hepatic and renal lesions. *CT* will demonstrate well-defined, rounded defects with an attenuation value close to 0 HU that is not modified after intravenous contrast material injection. In this case as well, the problem is differential diagnosis from parasitic cysts (Anjou et al. 1983; Solbiati et al. 1983).

4.2.1.3 False Cysts

False, or secondary cysts represent cystic degeneration of hematoma or infarction, and are fairly common. It has been estimated that there are four false cysts for every nonparasitic true cyst (Combe et al. 1980).

False cysts may appear calcified on *plain radiographs* (Sandermann 1981). Their *sonographic appearance* is the same as that of simple cysts: anechoic defects with smooth walls and posterior enhancement (Mittelstaedt and Partain 1980). *CT scans* will demonstrate a lesion with an attenuation value close to 0 HU which does not enhance (Anjou et al. 1983; Piekarski et al. 1980).

The clinical setting (elderly patient) and the patient's medical history (trauma, use of anticoagulant drugs) allow differentiation from parasitic cysts.

4.2.1.4 Enteroid Cysts

A recent entity first described by Issa et al. (1984), enteroid cysts occur late in life and apparently have a low propensity for malignant change. They cannot be differentiated from other benign cystic lesions using available imaging techniques. Surgery is the treatment of choice owing to a risk of rupture estimated at 20%.

4.2.2 Benign Noncystic Tumors

4.2.2.1 Hamartoma

Hamartoma, a rare benign splenic neoplasm, is often an incidental discovery at autopsy. These lymphoid tumors may be solitary or multiple; the cystic component predominates in hepatic sites. Hamartomas are usually asymptomatic, varying in size from several millimeters to several centimeters, although hypersplenism has been reported. The prognosis is favorable.

On *sonograms,* these inhomogeneous fluid-filled masses have a solid, more echogenic component than the normal spleen (Brinkley and Lee 1981). CT scans demonstrate a poorly demarcated solid lesion with a density identi-cal to that of the spleen, occasionally with a cystic component (Brinkley and Lee 1981; Ohta et al. 1986). *Angiograms* show a well-limited neovascularized mass with aneurysmal arterial dilatations and multiple vascular lakes. The splenic artery may be stretched by the mass. Similar findings have been reported for hemangiomas, hemangiosarcomas, and hematomas (Rosenthall et al. 1973). *Scintigraphy* is reportedly helpful for diagnosis owing to increased uptake of ^{51}chromium by lesions (Spalding et al. 1980).

4.2.2.2 Hemangioma (Figs. 4.31 to 4.33)

Hemangiomas account for 0.03%–14% of autopsy findings (Bevilacqua et al. 1976; Husni

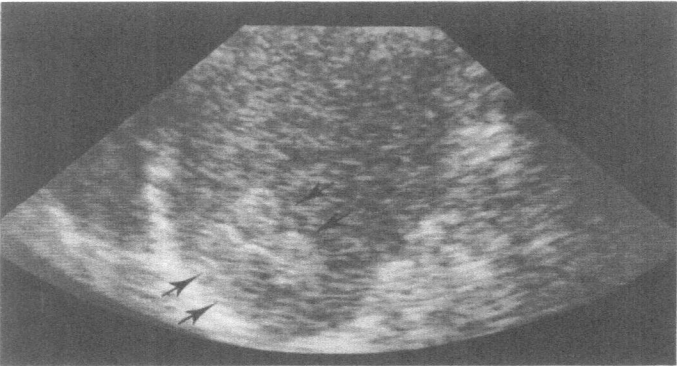

Fig. 4.31. Cavernous hemangioma: hyperechoic pattern (sagittal scan). (Courtesy of Dr. Matter)

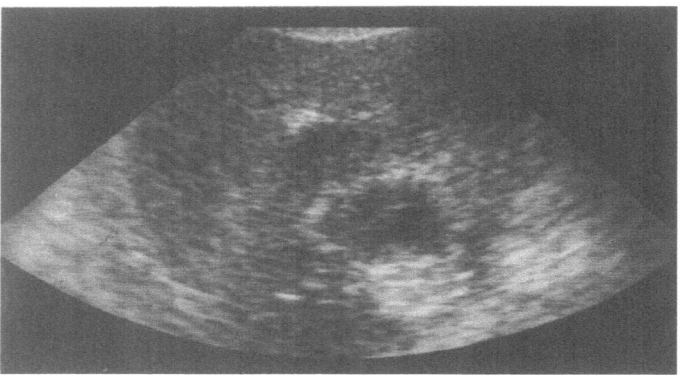

Fig. 4.32. Cavernous hemangioma: hypoechoic pattern (sagittal scan). (Courtesy of Dr. Matter)

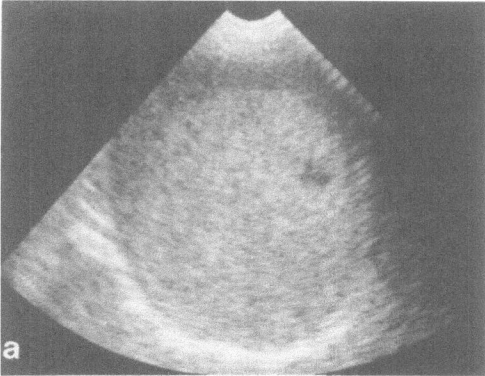

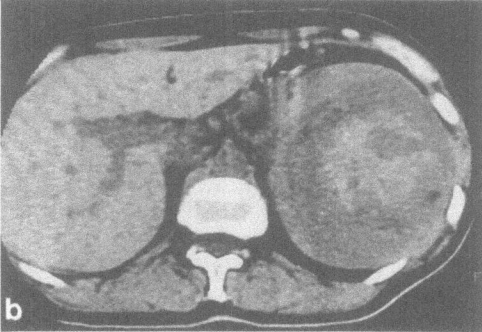

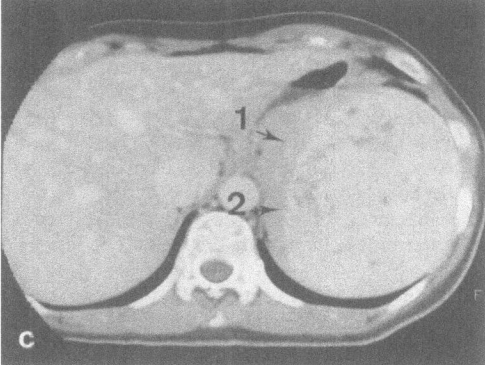

Fig. 4.33 a–c. Cavernous hemangioma: ultrasonography (sagittal scan) demonstrated a large hyperechoic homogeneous mass (**a**). On precontrast CT (**b**), the central part of the lesion showed increased density due to a central hemangioma. Late postcontrast CT (**c**) revealed a hyperdense lesion *(2)* stretching the normal parenchyma *(1)*

1961). Prior to the advent of ultrasonography, 30.4% of all hemangiomas were not discovered until necropsy. The major presenting feature of these often clinically latent tumors is patent splenomegaly. Symptoms are related to organ enlargement and subsequent compression of adjacent structures. Twenty-five percent of splenic hemangiomas are discovered after spontaneous rupture causing an acute abdominal emergency. The most frequent complications after rupture include hypersplenism, portal hypertension, and degeneration (Husni 1961).

Scintigraphy may reveal an intrasplenic filling defect (Leonard et al. 1981; Segal et al. 1977). Three *sonographic patterns* of splenic hemangioma have been identified: multiple, often confluent sonolucent nodules (cavernous hemangioma), solitary or multiple hyperechoic homogeneous nodules (capillary or cavernous hemangioma), and inhomogeneous hypoechoic defects (intratumoral infarcts; Manor et al. 1984).

CT may demonstrate calcifications, nonenhancing cystic lesions, or an isodense or hyperdense mass visible only after intravenous contrast infusion (Anjou et al. 1983; Balu-Maestro et al. 1986; Noya et al. 1984; Pakter et al. 1987).

Capillary hemangiomas may show up as hypervascular nodules on *arteriograms;* cavernous hemangiomas may present as multiple vascular lakes or an anarchic arterial distribution with incomplete parenchymal opacification in the late venous phases (Balu-Maestro et al. 1986; Kishikawa et al. 1978; Rosenthall et al. 1973).

Owing to the serious risks of malignant degeneration and hemorrhagic rupture, splenectomy is widely indicated for splenic hemangioma. Promising results have been obtained by embolization of the tumor's vascular pedicle (Noya et al. 1984).

4.2.2.3 Lymphangioma

Twenty percent of all nonparasitic true cysts of the spleen are cystic lymphangiomas. Not all splenic lymphangiomas are cystic however. The Landing and Farber classification (Pyatt et al. 1981) defines three categories: simple (capillary) lymphangiomas consisting of dilated lymph vessels; cavernous lymphangiomas formed by dilated lymphatic channels, often with a fibrous adventitial coat; and cystic lymphangiomas. The spleen is the least common site of cystic lymphangiomas (2%; Combe et al. 1980).

Most splenic lymphangiomas (80%) are moderate-sized unilocular subcapsular tumors; the remaining 20% are multilocular lesions which probably represent early stages of the disease. Children and adolescents account for 80% of all cases of splenic lymphangioma. Discovery of such a lesion should prompt a search for associated anomalies, and especially other lymphatic malformations and diffuse angiomatosis. These lesions are usually asymptomatic. Splenomegaly is a rare complication.

The *sonographic features* correspond to a transsonic cyst. Polycystic lymphangiomatosis of the spleen may be imaged as multiple cystic defects corresponding to the presence of septae (Combe et al. 1980; Mittelstaedt and Partain 1980). Splenic lymphangiomas have a *CT* density between 15 and 33 HU, similar to that of other processes with a fluid or necrotic component (Pyatt et al. 1981). *Arteriograms* demonstrate stretching of the intrasplenic arteries and an absence of vascular anomalies (Ellison 1980).

Ultrasound-guided biopsy allows accurate diagnosis (Combe et al. 1980). Despite the low risk of malignant transformation, progressive splenic enlargement suggests rupture, and is an indication for splenectomy (Combe et al. 1980; Rappaport 1966).

4.2.2.4 Other Benign Tumors

Splenic fibromas, myxomas, teratomas, and lipomas are extremely rare benign neoplasms, and have been excluded from this study (Anjou et al. 1983; Rappaport 1966).

4.3 Conclusion

Relatively few studies have compared ultrasonography and computed tomography for investigations of the spleen. In our experience, CT appears superior to ultrasound for the detection of small lesions in normal-sized spleens that are not always easy to explore sonographically; this is particularly true for splenic metastases. Evaluation of the dimensions of an enlarged spleen requires contact scanning, and the sonographic features of splenic tumors are often nonspecific. Sonographic detection of a splenic mass in an adult warrants complementary CT studies that may allow preoperative etiologic diagnosis. Even in patients without a recognized hematologic disease or primary cancer, surgery is often indicated owing to the risk of rupture associated with pathologic spleens.

4.4 References

Anjou A, Chollat L, Bret PM, Bretagnolle M, Valette PJ, Poix D (1983) Apport de la tomodensitométrie dans la pathologie splénique focalisée. Ann Radiol 26: 275-283

Arnold J, Mac Gahan JP, Stadalnick RC (1982) Epidermoid cyst of the spleen: value of non-invasive imaging modalities in preoperative diagnosis. J Comput Assist Tomogr 6: 836-838

Balu C, Bruneton JN, Fenart D, Nicolau A, Roux P, Caramella E (1984) Examen clinique et échographique. Valeur comparée dans l'exploration des masses de l'hypochondre gauche. Concours Médical 106: 2081-2086

Balu-Maestro C, Bruneton JN, Denis F, Fenart D, Abbes M, Normand F (1986) Hémangiome caverneux de la rate. J Radiol 67: 247-250

Bevilacqua G, Toni G, Tuoni M (1976) A case of cavernous hemangioma of the spleen. Tumori 62: 485-492

Bisker J, Mac Carthy J (1983) Computed tomographic demonstration of colonic carcinoma metastatic to the spleen. Comput Radiol 7: 193-194

Bostick WL (1945) Primary splenic neoplasms. Am J Path 21: 1143

Brinkley AA, Lee JR (1981) Cystic hamartoma of the spleen. CT and sonographic finding. J Clin Ultrasound 9: 136-138

Bruneton JN, Philippe JC, Balu C, Drouillard J, Caramella E, Roux P (1983) L'échographie en pathologie tumorale de la rate: limites et perspectives. Rev Fr Hématol 25: 355-361

Bruneton JN, Matter D, Benozio M, Senecail B (1984) Echographie en pathologie tumorale de l'adulte. Masson, Paris

Bruneton JN, Manzino JJ, Caramella E (1986) Gastrointestinal lymphomas. In: Bruneton JN, Schneider M (eds) Radiology of lymphomas. Springer, Berlin Heidelberg New York Tokyo, pp 70-89

Buf° SJ, Forster WL (1980) Left upper quadrant mass. Invest Radiol 15: 465–468

Carpenter G, Cotter PW, Davidson JRM (1986) Epidermoid cyst of the spleen. Aust NZ J Surg 56: 365–368

Combe J, Lorthioir JM, Muenier CL, Pageaut G, Dreyfus A, Millon G, Milleret P (1980) Lymphangiome kystique de la rate. J Chir 117: 547–550

Dawes LG, Malangoni MA (1986) Cystic masses of the spleen. Am Surg 52: 333–336

De Graaff CS, Taylor KJW, Jacobson Z (1979) Grey scale echography of the spleen. Follow-up in 67 patients. Ultrasound Med Biol 5: 13–21

Ellison RB (1980) Radiologic Seminar CCI: Cystic lymphangioma. A consideration in asymptomatic massive cystic splenomegaly. J Miss State Med Assoc 21: 67–68

Federle M, Moss AA (1983) Computed tomography of the spleen. CRC Crit Rev Diag Imaging 19: 1–16

Garcia Correa F, Febles Molina G, Perez Frias P, Alonso Gonzalez MA (1985) Quieste seroso del bazo. Rev Esp Enf Ap Digest 68: 162–165

Glees JP, Taylor KJW, Gazet JC, Peckham MJ, Mc Cready VR (1977) Accuracy of grey-scale ultrasonography of liver and spleen in Hodgkin's disease and the other lymphomas compared with isotope scans. Clin Radiol 28: 233–238

Goldfinger M, Cohen MM, Steinhardt MI, Rothberg R, Rother I (1986) Sonography and percutaneous aspiration of splenic epidermoid cyst. J Clin Ultrasound 14: 147–149

Husni EA (1961) The clinical course of splenic hemangioma. Arch Surg 83: 681–688

Issa M, Buemi A, Holderbach LJ, Ratignier A, Laedlein-Greilsamer D, Sengler J (1984) Kyste enteroïde de la rate: une nouvelle entité? J Chir 121: 425–429

Kishikawa T, Nymaguchi Y, Watanabe K, Matsuura K (1978) Angiographic diagnosis of benign and malignant splenic tumors. AJR 130: 339–344

Labbe A, Vanneuville G, Goomy P, Tanguy A, Viallet JF (1981) Kyste épidermoïde de la rate chez l'enfant. A propos d'une observation. Ann Radiol 24: 525–529

Leonard JC, Barnes PD, Kern JD (1981) Splenic hemangioma. Clin Nucl Med 6: 89

Lorenz R, Beyer D, Friedmann G, Mödder U (1983) Grenzen der Differenzierung fokaler Milzläsionen durch Sonographie und Computertomographie. RÖFO 138: 447–452

Manor A, Starinsky R, Garfinkel D, Yona E, Modai D (1984) Ultrasound features of a symptomatic splenic hemangioma. J Clin Ultrasound 12: 95–97

Meyer JE, Harris NL, Elman A, Stomper PC (1983) Large cell lymphoma of the spleen: CT appearance. Radiology 148: 199–201

Mittelstaedt CA, Partain CL (1980) Ultrasonic-pathologic classification of splenic abnormalities: gray scale patterns. Radiology 134: 697–705

Murphy JF, Bernardino ME (1979) The sonographic findings of splenic metastases. J Clin Ultrasound 7: 195–197

Nahman B, Cunningham JJ (1985) Sonography of splenic angiosarcoma. J Clin Ultrasound 13: 354–356

Newmark H (1982) Breast cancer metastasizing to the spleen seen on computerized tomography. Comput Radiol 6: 53–55

Noya G, Riberti C, Dettori G, Bacciu PP, Sala A, Gauisai D, Urigo F, Bigglioli P (1984) L'emangioma cavernose splenico. Minerva Med 75: 483–486

Ohta M, Tsutsumi Y, Tanaka Y (1986) Splenic hamartoma. Acta Pathol Jpn 36: 471–480

Pakter RL, Fishman EK, Nussbaum A, Giargiana FA, Zerhouni EA (1987) CT findings in splenic hemangiomas in the Klippel-Trenaunay-Weber-Syndrome. J Comput Assist Tomogr 11: 88–91

Piekarski J, Federle MP, Moss AA, London SS (1980) Computed tomography of the spleen. Radiology 135: 683–689

Pyatt RS, Williams ED, Clark M, Gaskins R (1981) CT diagnosis of splenic cyst lymphangiomatosis. J Comput Assist Tomogr 5: 446–448

Quilichini MA, Clot P, Viandier A, Gayet B, Douard MC, Vaquino G (1983) Kyste épidermoïde de la rate. A propos de 2 cas. Ann Chir 37: 341–344

Rappaport H (1966) Tumors of the hematopoietic system. Atlas of tumor pathology, Sect III, Fasc 8. AFIP, Washington, pp 91–204

Rosenthall T, Adar R, Wolfstein I, Deutsch V (1973) Cavernous hemangioma of the spleen; angiographic observations. Angiology 24: 430–433

Sandermann J (1981) Secondary calcified splenic cyst. Acta Chir Scand 147: 725–727

Segal I, Fancourt MN, Kecker GAG, Hodgkinson JH (1977) Cavernous hemangioma of the spleen. A case report. J South Afr Med Assoc 51: 637–638

Sekiya T, Meller ST, Cosgrove O, Mac Ready VR (1982) Ultrasonography of Hodgkin's disease in the liver and spleen. Clin Radiol 33: 635–639

Siler J, Hunter TB, Weiss J, Haber K (1980) Increased echogenicity of the spleen in benign and malignant disease. AJR 134: 1011–1014

Solbiati L, Bossi MC, Bellotto E, Ravetto C, Montali G (1983) Focal lesions in the spleen. Sonographic patterns and guided biopsy. AJR 140: 59–65

Spalding RM, Jennings CU, Yam LT (1980) Splenic hamartoma. Br J Radiol 53: 1197–1200

Thomas JL, Bernardino ME, Vermess M, Bernes PA, Fuller LM, Hagemeister FB, Doppman J, Fisher RI, Longo DL (1982) EOE-13 in the detection of hepatosplenic lymphoma. Radiology 145: 629–634

Tran-Minh V, Pichat L, Giuy J, Valla JS, Mollard P (1980) Kyste épidermoïde de la rate. Signe échographique inhabituel. Ann Radiol 23: 429–430

Vermess M, Bernardino ME, Doppmann JL, Fisher RI, Thomas JL, Velasquez WS, Fuller LM, Russo A (1981) Use of intravenous liposoluble contrast material for the examination of the liver and spleen in lymphoma. J Comput Assist Tomogr 5: 700-713

Vermess M, Doppmann JL, Sugarbaker PH, Fisher RI, O'Leary TS, Chatterji DC, Grimes G, Adamson RH, Willis M, Edwards BK (1982) Computed tomography of the liver and spleen with intravenous lipoid contrast material: review of 60 examinations. AJR 138: 1063-1071

Zornoza J, Ginaldi S (1981) Computed tomography in hepatic lymphoma. Radiology 138: 405-410

5 Splenic Abscess and Infarction

C. ANAGNOSTOUPOULOS, P. JACQUENOD, S. CHAGNON, M. BLÉRY

Splenic abscess is an unusual entity with an incidence of only 0.14%–0.70% in large autopsy series. Altemeier et al. (1973), for example, failed to find any cases in their review of 540 intraabdominal abscesses. The rarity of splenic infections can be explained by this organ's phagocytic activity and its role in the immune system, which give it a unique capacity to resist local infection (Sarr and Zuidema 1982). As early as 1938, Caldarera suggested that both an infectious agent (reaching the spleen by hematogenous spread or direct contact with a local focus of infection) and a pathologic spleen (defective function or architecture) are required to initiate splenic abscess.

5.1 Pathogenesis

Splenic abscess can occur as the result of hematogenous seeding of bacteria from an infection elsewhere in the body or direct extension of infection in a contiguous organ.

5.1.1 Hematogenous Spread

Hematogenous spread of bacteria is the most frequent cause of splenic abscess (80% of cases). *Bacterial endocarditis* is the most common etiology (Epstein and Omar 1983). Owing to the end-arterial nature of the splenic vasculature (Chun et al. 1980), embolic occlusion can lead to infarction. A septic embolus will cause abscess formation from the outset; an infarct caused by a sterile embolus may become superinfected ulteriorly by hematogenous spread of bacteria.
Hemolytic anemia, and especially heterozygous sickle-cell disease, is accompanied by multiple splenic infarcts susceptible to infection (Johnson et al. 1983).

Immunosuppression is another predisposing factor. Heroin addicts are especially susceptible to splenic abscess as they are both immunocompromised and present multiple pathways for infection. Patients treated with antimitotics and immunosuppressants are also at risk for splenic abscess, as are individuals with congenital immune system dysfunction (Freund et al. 1982).

5.1.2 Direct Extension of a Local Infection

Superinfection of a posttraumatic splenic hematoma accounts for 15% of all splenic abscesses (Dupuy et al. 1984; Fry et al. 1978). Preexisting splenic cysts and pancreatic pseudocysts are also subject to superinfection and abscess formation (Magid et al. 1984; Ralls et al. 1982; Soderstrom 1979). By contrast, visualization of air bubbles in the spleen after therapeutic embolization does not necessarily indicate infection: such images may merely reflect simple necrosis. Neoplastic disease in a contiguous organ (colon, stomach) is a less frequent predisposing factor.

5.1.3 Bacteriology

A wide range of pathogens cause splenic abscess: there is no predominant organism. Severe splenic mycoses (with *Candida* or *Aspergillus*) have been reported in immunocompromised patients (Berlow et al. 1984; Freund et al. 1982; Linos et al. 1983; Miller et al. 1982).

5.2 Clinical Presentation

Presenting symptoms associated with splenic abscess are variable, and may develop several days to several months before diagnosis. The mean duration of symptoms is 22 days. The patient generally presents with generalized sepsis (deteriorated clinical status and fever). Pain and left upper quadrant tenderness may suggest the diagnosis, but some patients have only mild abdominal complaints or even no abdominal symptoms at all. White blood cell studies usually reveal a large number of polymorphonuclear leukocytes.

5.3 Imaging Studies

5.3.1 Chest Radiographs

Chest radiographs may demonstrate left pleural effusion or left lower lobe atelectasis. Abdominal plain films occasionally demonstrate splenomegaly.

5.3.2 Ultrasonography and Computed Tomography

Ultrasonography and computed tomography can both demonstrate parenchymal abnormalities suggestive of splenic abscess. Use of these techniques is particularly indicated for examination of patients with vague complaints in whom the only symptoms may be a prolonged febrile course, without any specific physical findings (Inlow 1927; Miller et al. 1982).

5.3.2.1 Ultrasonography

Splenic abscesses present a variety of sonographic patterns (Miller et al. 1982; Morgenstern et al. 1984; Figs. 5.1 to 5.4):

- Relatively complex hypoechoic or hyperechoic focal lesions, sometimes with posterior reinforcement. Dense echoes with an acoustic shadow correspond to the presence of air.
- A well-delimited mass or several poorly defined masses of variable size; splenomegaly is inconstant
- A triangular image with the base at the splenic capsule, typical of splenic infarcts

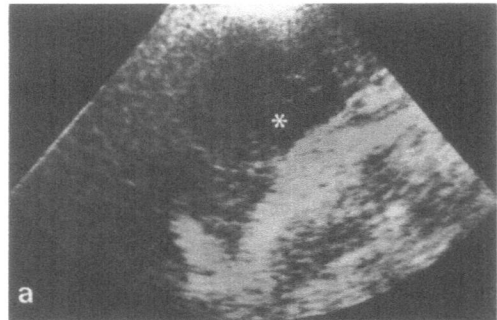

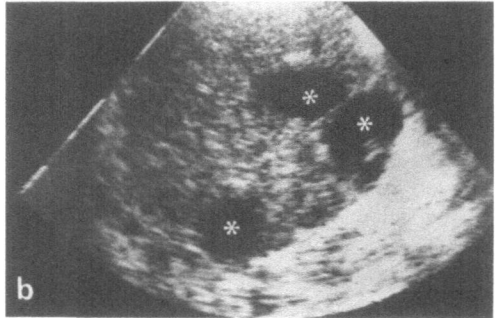

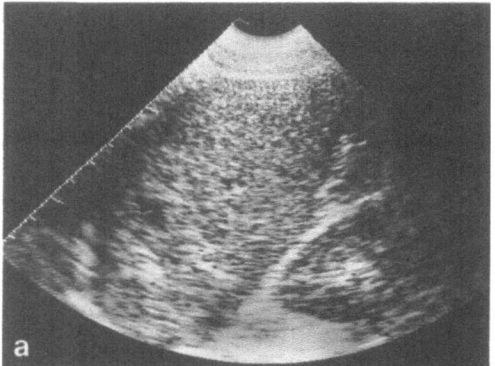

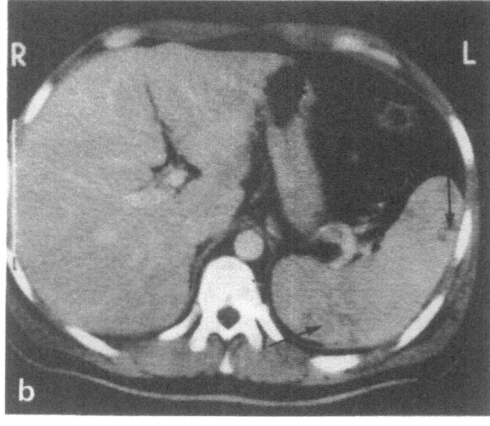

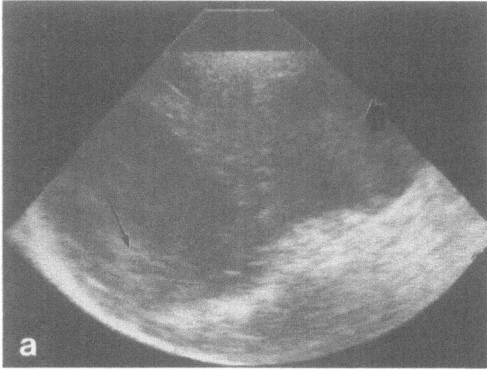

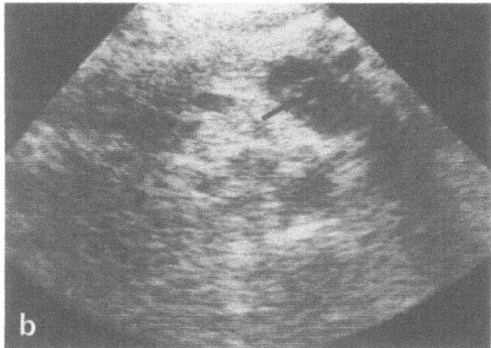

Fig.5.3a, b. 54-year-old woman with isolated fever. Splenic sonogram **a**: heterogeneous splenomegaly with hyperechoic *(thin arrow)* and hypoechoic *(thick arrow)* zones, with irregular contours, corresponding to an infarcted spleen with abscesses and splenic rupture several days later, where **b** ultrasonography demonstrated a poorly defined heterogeneous collection in the celiomesenteric and perisplenic region *(arrow)*

◄ **Fig.5.1** *(above).* **a** 81-year-old woman with angiocholitis and splenic and hepatic abscesses. Splenic sonogram: normal size spleen with a hypoechoic collection greater than 3 cm. **b** Hepatic sonogram: multiple hypoechoic zones with posterior reinforcement and irregular contours (*)

Fig. 5.2a, b *(below).* 36-year-old man with ankylosing spondylarthritis and fever. Splenic ultrasonography revealed multiple abscesses smaller than 2 cm *(arrow)* (**a**). CT appearance (**b**): multiple hypodense zones of variable size at the periphery, with irregular contours *(arrows)*

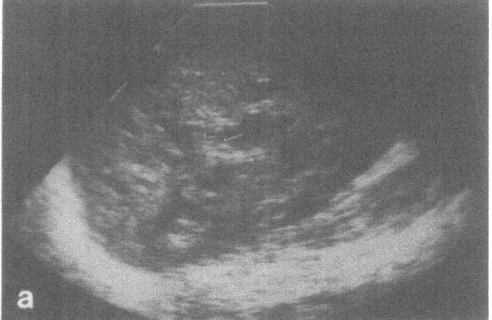

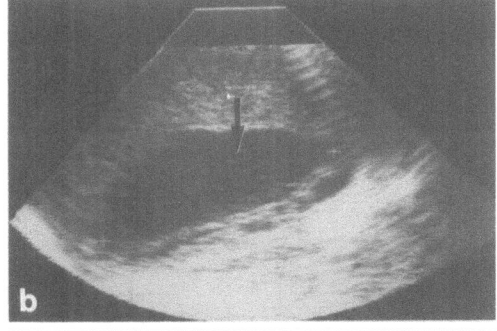

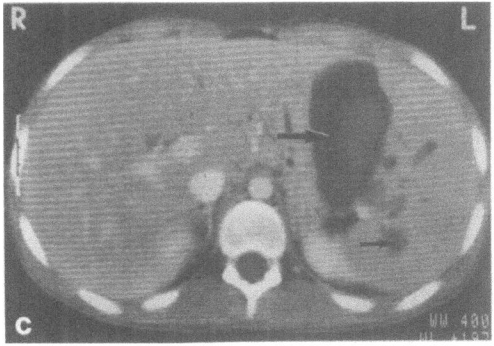

Fig.5.4a-c. Multiple splenic abscesses in a heroin addict. First splenic sonogram **a**: splenomegaly with several small (less than 2 cm), irregular hypoechoic zones. Second splenic sonogram 1 week later (**b**) rupture of a splenic abscess was visualized as a hypoechoic collection with internal debris located along the internal border of the spleen (*arrow;* 6 cm between the two *crosses*). CT examination (**c**) the same day as **b**: abscess with irregular contours less than 2 cm (intrasplenic areas of hypodensity; *small arrow*) and a subcapsular collection (hypodense and slightly heterogeneous; *large arrow*)

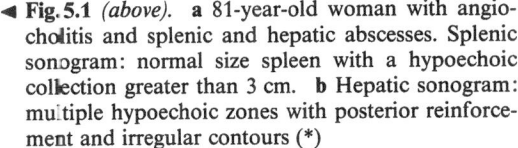

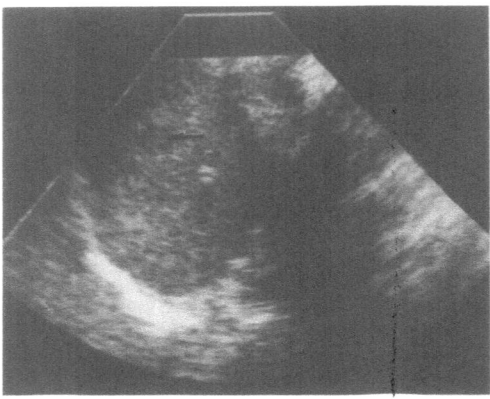

Fig. 5.5. Tuberculous abscess: rounded hypoechoic defect (2 cm between the two *crosses*)

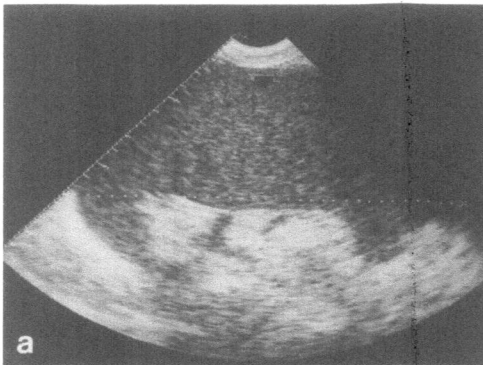

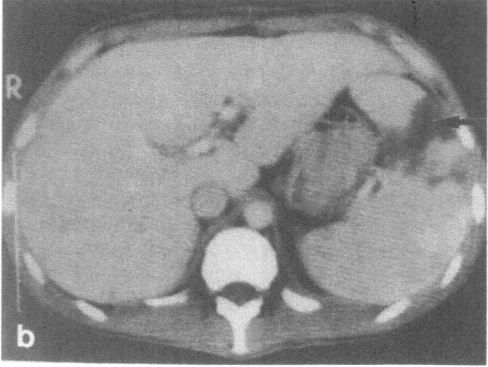

Fig. 5.6a, b. 35-year-old man with bacterial endocarditis and splenic infarcts. **a** Splenic sonogram: homogeneous splenomegaly *(thick arrow).* **b** CT scan: demonstration of several hypodense zones at the periphery with their base towards the capsule *(thin arrow),* corresponding to splenic infarcts. This was a case of discordance between US and CT

Splenic abscesses may be associated with numerous other lesions: perisplenic collections, intraperitoneal effusions or multiple abscesses, particularly in the liver. In one personal observation, a tuberculous splenic abscess was accompanied by celiomesenteric adenopathies (Fig. 5.5). However, drug addicts with AIDS also have a high incidence of adenopathies, and thorough examinations of the spleen is indispensable.

5.3.2.2 Computed Tomography (CT)

Postcontrast CT scans demonstrate splenic abscesses as low density lesions (Anjou et al. 1983; Balthazar et al. 1985; Berlow et al. 1984; Moreaux and Bismuth 1969); contours may appear rounded or irregular. Both solitary and multiple lesions may occur. We, ourselves, have never encountered the "bull's-eye" pattern described for hepatic abscesses. Occasionally, the CT appearance is suggestive of splenic infarction: a wedge-shaped defect at the periphery of the organ or a massive hypodense defect that may occupy almost the entire spleen (Balcar et al. 1984). Slight peripheral enhancement is possible. The splenic vasculature may not be affected (Cohen et al. 1984). CT is an excellent technique for localizing subcapsular and perisplenic fluid collections (Balthazar et al. 1985). In those rare instances that the splenic parenchyma appears sonographically normal, CT will demonstrate extensive infarction (Fig. 5.6). Such discordance between sonographic and CT findings suggests infarction, because it is our experience that splenic abscesses are always correctly diagnosed by ultrasound.

5.4 Differential Diagnosis

Apart from the typical wedge-shaped appearance of infarcts, there are no specific sonographic or CT signs diagnostic for splenic abscess. The main goal of such imaging techniques is identification of splenic involvement; findings must always be interpreted in light of the clinical context. Major differential diagnoses include:

- Splenic hematoma and contusion: in advanced stages, these lesions image similarly to splenic abscesses, but there is a history of trauma and no infectious syndrome (although superinfection is possible).
- Epidermoid or posttraumatic splenic cysts: asymptomatic unless very large, cysts of this type have a smooth contour; they generally contain fluid, and may show septations. Superinfection is again a possibility.
- Solid lesions: splenic sites of hematologic disorders, metastasis, rare benign tumors (hamartoma; Brinkley and Lee 1981; Manor et al. 1984).
- Parasitic lesions and hydatid cysts: the clinical setting and blood tests should allow correct diagnosis.
- Angioma: diagnosis can be made by CT performed with rapid contrast medium injection (Laurin and Kaude 1984).

When doubt persists, diagnostic percutaneous thin-needle aspiration has been recommended, especially as there is no risk of complications (Balcar et al. 1984; Rao et al. 1981; Sarr and Zuidema 1982; Schwerk et al. 1986; Sitzmann and Imbembo 1984).

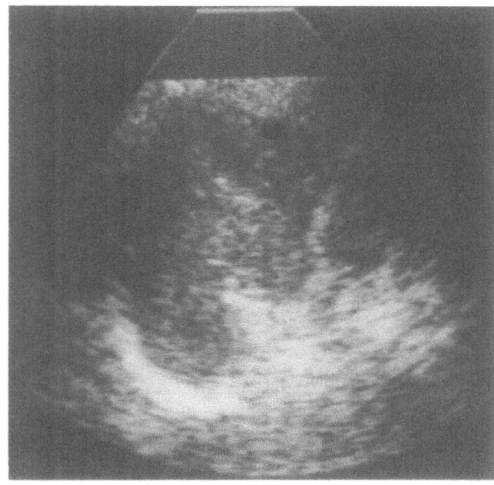

Fig. 5.7. 63-year-old man with bacterial endocarditis. Splenic sonogram: hypoechoic zones with irregular contours *(arrow)* corresponding to several small splenic abscesses. Administration of antibiotics led to complete disappearance of all lesions in 3 weeks

5.5 Relation Between Splenic Abscess and Infarction

The classical belief that an abscess requires surgery while an infarct can be managed medically has come under attack (Hart et al. 1969). In fact, splenic infarcts can evolve with time, transforming into an abscess following superinfection. Abscess and infarct can thus be considered the two extremes of a wide range of situations (Balthazar et al. 1985).

5.6 Conclusion

Sonographically demonstrated splenic lesions can usefully be classified in two categories. *Extensive* lesions associated with fluid collections: operative mortality rises from 10% to 40% when complications such as perisplenic or intraperitoneal rupture or portal thrombosis occur (Chulay and Lankeran 1976). Such lesions are lethal in the absence of surgery. Even when surgery is performed, the prognosis depends on the rapidity of intervention and the subjacent terrain. Splenectomy with appropriate antibiotic coverage is the standard treatment, but the procedure can be complicated by the presence of numerous inflammatory adherences.

Small (less than 2 cm) solitary or multiple splenic lesions may completely disappear with adequate antibiotic treatment: this can be confirmed by follow-up CT and ultrasound scans (Anjou et al. 1983; Figs. 5.7 and 5.8). Both Balthazar et al. (1985) and Linos et al. (1983) have reported an increase in the rate of detection of such small lesions. This situation can be explained by the improved performances of imaging techniques, which today locate previously undetectable splenic abnormalities. The incidence of occult splenic abscesses which disappear with antibiotic treatment, as in infectious endocarditis, for example, is also probably underestimated (Chun et al. 1980; Hart et al. 1969).

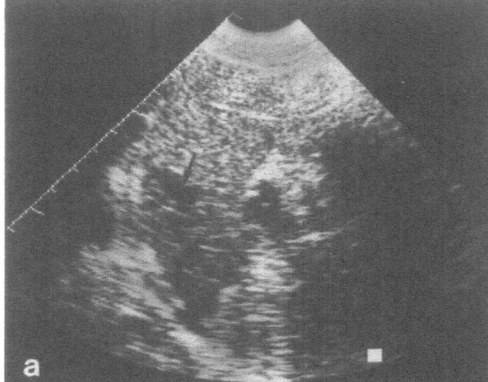

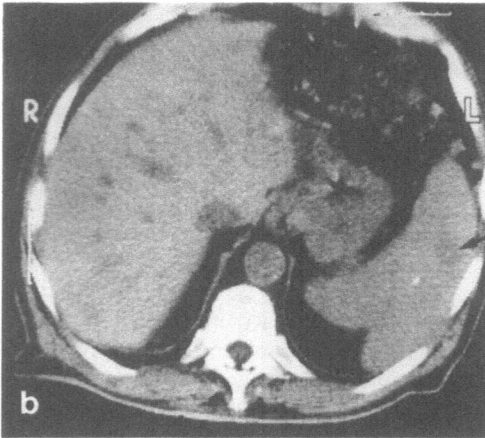

Fig. 5.8 a, b. 88-year-old man with a urinary infection. **a** Sonogram: hypoechoic zone with irregular contours smaller than 2 cm *(arrow).* **b** CT scan: hypodense defect *(arrow).* The diagnosis was intrasplenic abscess. Return to normal after administration of antibiotics

5.7 References

Altemeier WA, Culbertson WR, Fullen WD, Shook CD (1973) Intra-abdominal abscesses. Am J Surg 125: 70–79

Anjou A, Chollat L, Bret PM, Bretagnolle M, Valetta PJ, Poix D (1983) Apport de la tomodensitométrie dans la pathologie splénique focalisée. Ann Radiol 26: 275–283

Balcar I, Seltzer SE, Davis S, Geller S (1984) CT patterns of splenic infarction: a clinical and experimental study. Radiology 151: 723–729

Balthazar EJ, Hilton S, Naidich D, Megibow A, Levine R (1985) CT of splenic and perisplenic abnormalities in septic patients. AJR 144: 53–56

Berlow ME, Spirt BA, Weil L (1984) CT follow-up of hepatic and splenic fungal microabscesses. J Comput Assist Tomogr 8: 45

Brinkley AA, Lee JKT (1981) Cystic hamartoma of the spleen. CT and sonographic findings. J Clin Ultrasound 9: 136–138

Caldarera E (1938) Acute abscess of the spleen. Surg Gynecol 67: 265

Chulay JD, Lankeran MR (1976) Splenic abscess: report of 10 cases and review of the literature. Am J Med 61: 513–522

Chun CH, Raff MJ, Contreras L, Varghese R, Waterman N, Daffner R, Melo JC (1980) Splenic abscess. Medicine 59: 50–65

Cohen BA, Mitty HA, Mendelson DS (1984) Computed tomography of splenic infarction. J Comput Assist Tomogr 8: 167–168

Dupuy JP, Catanzano G, Bouchet DB, Le Goff J (1984) Le lymphangiome kystique hépatosplénique. Ann Radiol 27: 417–420

Epstein BM, Omar GM (1983) Infective complications of splenic trauma. Clin Radiol 34: 91–94

Freund R, Pichl J, Heyder N, Rödl W, Riemann JF (1982) Splenic abscess – clinical symptoms and diagnostic possibilities. Am J Gastroent 77: 35–38

Fry DE, Richardson JD, Flint LM (1978) Occult splenic abscess: an unrecognized complication of heroin abuse. Surgery 84: 650–654

Hart PD, Russell E Jr, Remington JS (1969) The compromised host and infection. II. Deep fungal infection. J Infect is 120: 169–191

Inlow W de P (1927) Traumatic abscess of the spleen. Ann Surgery 85: 368–379

Johnson D, Raff MJ, Barnwell PL, Chun CH (1983) Splenic abscess complicating infectious endocarditis. Arch Int Med 143: 906–912

Laurin S, Kaude JV (1984) Diagnosis of liver-spleen abscesses in children with emphasis on ultrasound for the initial and follow-up examinations. Pediatr Radiol 14: 198–204

Linos DA, Nagorney DM, McIlrath DC (1983) Splenic abscess – the importance of early diagnosis. Mayo Clin Proc 58: 261–264

Magid D, Fishman EK, Siegelman SS (1984) Computed tomography of the spleen and liver in sickle cell disease. AJR 143: 245–249

Manor A, Starinsky R, Garfinkel D, Yona E, Modai D (1984) Ultrasound features of a symptomatic splenic hemangioma. J Clin Ultrasound 12: 95–97

Miller JH, Greenfield LD, Wald BR (1982) Candidiasis of the liver and spleen in childhood. Radiology 142: 375–380

Moreaux J, Bismuth H (1969) Les complications spléniques des pancréatites chroniques. A propos de 5 observations. Presse Med 77: 1467–1470

Morgenstern L, McCafferty L, Rosenberg J, Michel SL (1984) Hamartomas of the spleen. Arch Surg 119: 1291–1293

Ralls PW, Quinn MF, Colletti P, Lapin SA, Halls J (1982) Sonography of pyogenic splenic abscess. AJR 138: 523–525

Rao BK, Aubuchon J, Lieberman LM, Polcyn RE (1981) Cystic lymphangiomatosis of the spleen: a radiologic-pathologic correlation. Radiology 141: 781–782

Sarr MG, Zuidema GD (1982) Splenic abscess – presentation, diagnosis and treatment. Surgery 92: 480–485

Schwerk WB, Maroske D, Roth S, Arnold R (1986) Ultraschall-geführte Feinnadelpunktionen in der Diagnostik und Therapie von Leber und Milzabszessen. Dtsch Med Wochenschr 22: 847–853

Sitzmann JV, Imbembo AL (1984) Splenic complications of a pancreatic pseudocyst. Am J Surg 147: 191–196

Söderström N (1979) Cytology of the spleen. In: Zajicek J (ed) Aspiration biopsy cytology. Part 2. Cytology of infradiaphragmatic organs. Karger, Basel, pp 229–247

6 Splenic Involvement in Parasitoses

H. A. GHARBI, P. MARBOT, M. BEN CHEIKH

A sponge-like mass of reticuloendothelial tissue, the spleen is located upstream of the hepatic portal system and is supplied by a large artery: this makes the organ particularly susceptible to parasitic infections. Certain parasites infest the spleen itself, while others attack the hepatic structures, leading to secondary splenic venous stasis. The splenomegaly that frequently accompanies parasitic infections reflects the body's immune response to such insults (Wyler 1983).

Splenic lesions in parasitoses vary considerably, depending on the parasite and the degree and duration of infestation. Three basic types of involvement can be distinguished:

- The spleen itself is the site of parasitic lesions. In most cases, the parasite reaches the splenic parenchyma as the result of arterial hematogenous spread; once there, it establishes itself and undergoes development: the prime example is splenic hydatid disease. Ultrasonography is especially indicated in such cases as visualization of the typical cystic images will suggest the diagnosis.
- Splenic involvement is secondary to a "mechanical" obstacle downstream of the splenic vein causing portal hypertension. Schistosomiasis is the major example. Along with diagnosing portal hypertension, ultrasonography can suggest the etiology and evaluate the extent of damage.
- The spleen is involved as part of the body's general immune reaction to a parasitic infection. The typical example is malaria, with splenomegaly being the main clinical manifestation.

In addition to these three basic types of splenic involvement in parasitoses, there are numerous complex situations corresponding to intermediate disease stages.

The sonographic images of parasitic spleens range from a few rare pathognomonic signs to generally nonspecific patterns which cannot be interpreted correctly without reference to the clinical context, biological tests, and existence of an endemic situation. Nevertheless, ultrasonography remains particularly valuable: along with confirming the existence of splenic involvement and assessing relevant parameters (lesion size, margins, echo pattern, etc.), the technique can evaluate response to medical treatment or surgery and guide puncture biopsies. Ultrasonography is also an excellent means for diagnosing postoperative complications, especially infection, and for detecting associated parasitic lesions in other viscera.

Before detailing several parasitic diseases affecting the spleen, a word is warranted concerning equipment selection. Electronic scanning units seem best suited to systemic screening of populations in countries where parasitoses reach endemic proportions. Use of portable, easily serviced, and reliable equipment of this type facilitates work in the rural areas of many developing nations. As an example, we employed a linear scanner to conduct over 10 000 examinations in a 30-month-period at rural schools, factories, marketplaces, and other sites without any maintenance problems. In our experience, the quality of splenic examinations with such equipment is acceptable in over 95% of cases.

6.1 Parasitic Infections of the Spleen

6.1.1 Echinococcosis (Hydatid Disease)

6.1.1.1 Unilocular Hydatid Disease

Caused by *Echinococcus granulosis,* this cesto-diasis of cosmopolitan distribution occurs predominantly in areas of intensive sheep or cattle farming (Matossian et al. 1977).

General Features. Man is an accidental host in this animal parasitosis which involves two hosts: a definitive, carnivorous host (usually a dog) and an intermediate, herbivorous animal (sheep, cattle, camel).

The adult tapeworm lives in the jejunum of the dog; the eggs it releases are passed in the excreta. When ingested by an intermediate host, eggs reach the stomach and free embryos, which penetrate the intestinal wall and reach the liver through the portal system.

The larvae are carried to the lungs, and escape into the general circulation: no part of the organism is protected from infestation. The larvae rapidly become surrounded by an inflammatory granuloma and transform into a multinuclear protoplasmic mass which develops over a week into a vesicle or hydatid. Over a period of 16 to 20 weeks, the cyst doubles in size as it becomes filled with fluid. This period of progressive development leads to the production of thousands of scolices; at the same time, an intense tissue reaction around the vesicle results in formation of a tough wall called the pericyst.

If the intermediate, herbivorous host dies and cyst-containing flesh is eaten by a dog, each scolex grows to an adult worm in the jejunum. Like intermediate hosts, man becomes infected more often during close contact with dogs (hands licked by an infected animal, or hands brought in contact with the mouth after having touched an infected dog) than after ingestion of food or water contaminated by the excreta of infected dogs.

The geographic distribution of hydatid disease reflects the nature of the life cycle: the disease is endemic in rural areas where sheep and cattle are raised with the help of dogs (South America, Australia, New Zealand, East and especially North Africa, and around the Mediterranean).

Certain professions are particularly exposed to the risk of contracting hydatidosis: shepherds and sheep farmers, veterinarians and laboratory personnel, butchers and meat packers.

While all of the viscera may be affected, the liver and the lungs are the sites of predilection (respectively, two-thirds and one-fifth of all cases), followed by the kidney and the spleen (Gharbi et al. 1985; Horchani et al. 1983). The majority of splenic lesions are primary in nature, following arterial dissemination of the parasite through the hepatic and pulmonary tissues, which are not necessarily infested during the process.

Although the incidence of splenic hydatid disease is hard to determine, it has been estimated at 1%–5% of all cases of hydatidosis (Gharbi et al. 1985). There is no sex predilection, and infestation can occur at any age, generally from 2 years onwards. However, most cases are seen in young adults.

The clinical manifestations of splenic hydatidosis are variable, but generally include either a left upper quadrant mass or left upper quadrant pain. Diagnosis may result from an incidental finding during ultrasonography or discovery of a calcification on a plain abdominal film. On rare occasions, rupture of a cyst or compression of neighboring viscera prompts diagnosis.

Sonographic Features. The well-known sonographic features of abdominal hydatid cysts are also applicable to splenic lesions (Lewall and McCorkell 1985; De Dios-Vega et al. 1977; Gharbi et al. 1981; Hassine et al. 1980; King 1973; Weill 1980). Five sonographic patterns have been identified, corresponding to the various developmental stages of the hydatid cyst.

Type I: Simple Fluid Collection (Figs. 6.1 to 6.3). Imaged as rounded anechoic defects with marked enhancement of back wall echoes, pure fluid collections always have well-defined margins. Localized wall thickening is common; this feature should be sought systematically since it strongly suggests a hydatid cyst. Cysts at the periphery of the spleen, in contact with the abdominal wall or the diaphragm, may appear oval rather than rounded, and molded to the parietal contours.

Cyst size is extremely variable, ranging from 1 cm to over 15 cm in diameter. The most frequent sonographic pattern observed in the spleen, and especially in children, pure fluid collections correspond to young, uncomplicated, monovesicular cysts containing clear fluid. The differential diagnosis is easy, as only epidermoid cysts, pseudocystic hematomas, and pancreatic pseudocysts have similar appearances (Fig. 6.4). Epidemiological surveys, bio-

logical tests, and searches for associated hydatid lesions (particularly in the liver and lungs) can guide diagnosis.

Type II: Fluid Collection with a "Split Wall" (Figs. 6.5 and 6.6). These fluid collections also have well-defined contours, but are often less rounded than type I lesions. The cyst wall may appear to "sag" at certain points: this "split wall" appearance may be localized to a small

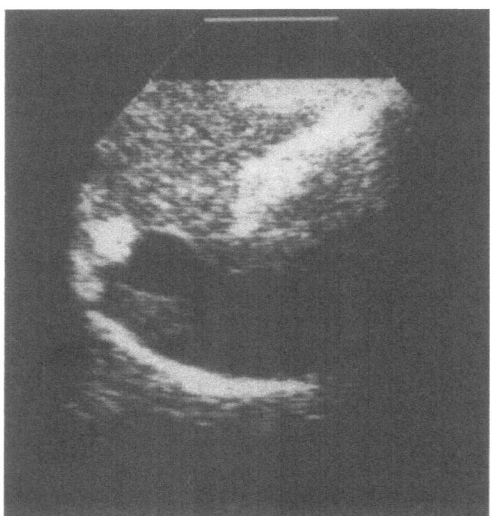

Fig. 6.1. 3-year-old child: 2 cm diameter splenic hydatid cyst (type I)

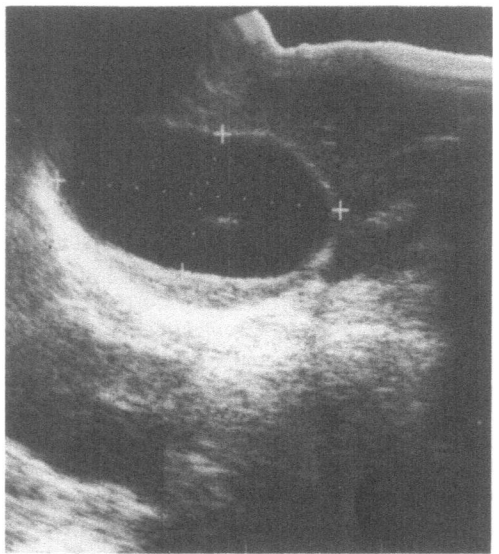

Fig. 6.2. 12-year-old girl: splenic hydatid cyst with a discretely thickened wall (17 cm in long axis)

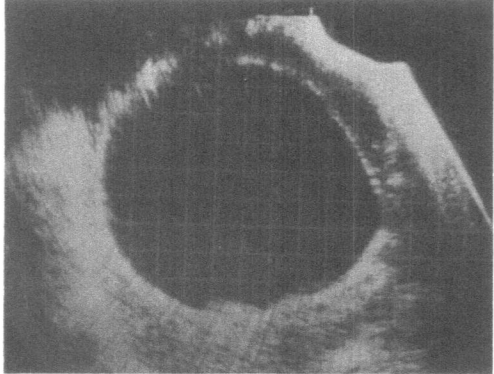

Fig. 6.3. Hydatid cyst (13 cm diameter) in an adult: type I

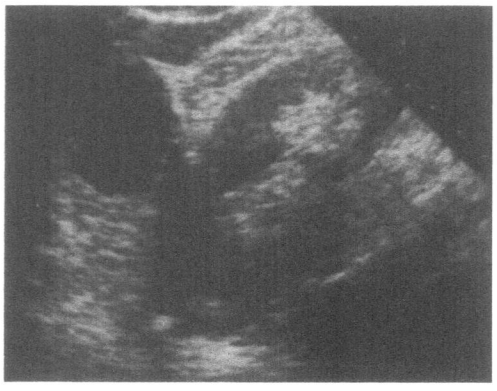

Fig. 6.4. Uncomplicated asymptomatic epidermoid cyst (4 cm diameter) discovered incidentally in a 46-year-old man

area on the periphery of the cyst or the membrane may be completely separate and float free within the cyst. All intrasplenic fluid collections must be systematically examined for this "split wall" image which is almost pathognomonic for hydatid cysts.

Type III: Septated Fluid Collection (Figs. 6.7 and 6.8). Type III lesions still have sharply defined margins, but are subdivided into oval or rounded compartments by complete septae of variable thickness. Back wall echoes are not always strongly enhanced. The most typical

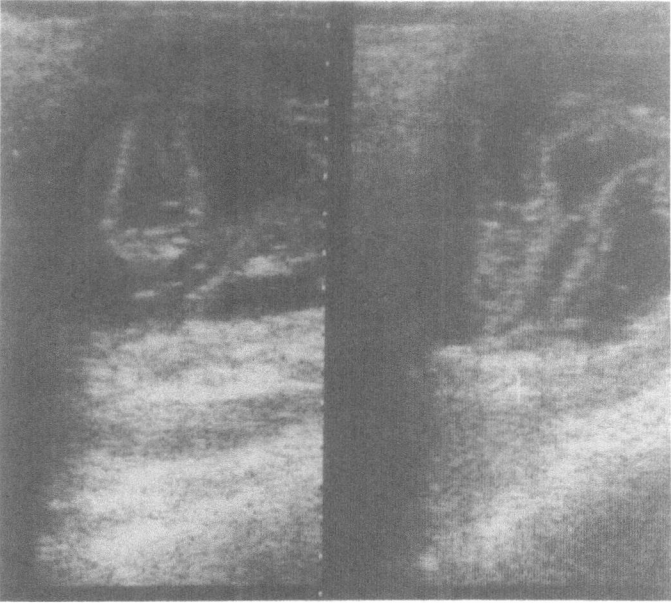

Fig. 6.5. Hydatid cyst in an 8-year-old girl: type II. Note the membrane that has separated completely and appears folded within the cyst

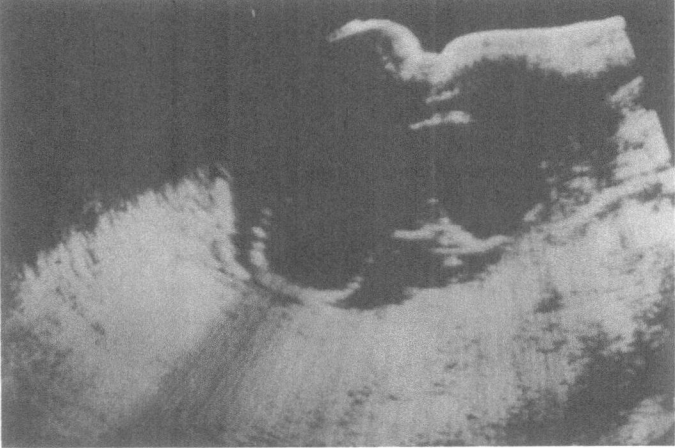

Fig. 6.6. Hydatid cyst in a 14-year-old girl: type II

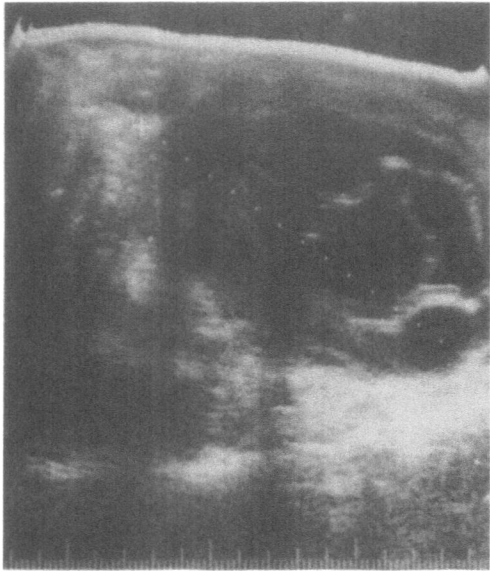

Fig. 6.7. Hydatid cyst in an 8-year-old girl: type III. Note the daughter vesicles and the separated membrane in the anterior spleen

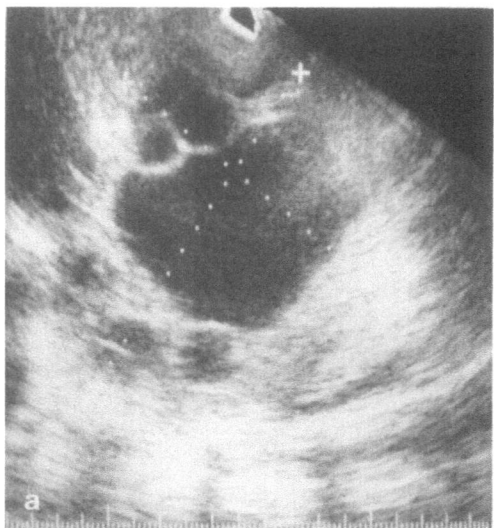

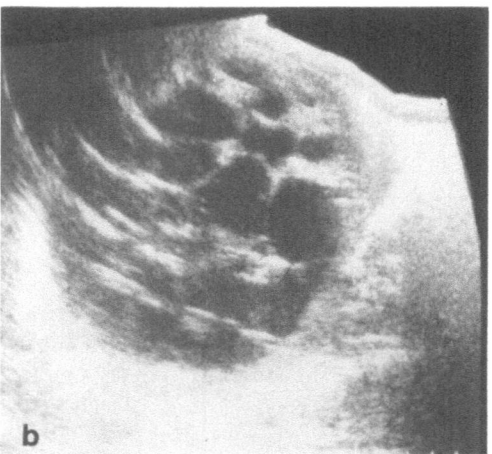

▶

Fig. 6.8 a, b. Large splenic hydatid cyst in a 45-year-old woman: type III

cases present a characteristic "honeycomb" image reflecting the presence of numerous intracystic secondary vesicles. Occasionally, a separated, folded cystic membrane will simulate the existence of several intracystic daughter vesicles. Such patterns are strongly suggestive of the diagnosis. Septated fluid collections are also seen in connection with cystic lymphangioma, but clinical data and biological tests can correct the diagnosis (Dupuy et al. 1984; Rao et al. 1981).

Type IV: Inhomogeneous Echo Pattern (Figs. 6.9 to 6.13). Lesions of this type are demonstrated as roughly rounded masses with irregular contours and a complex echo pattern.

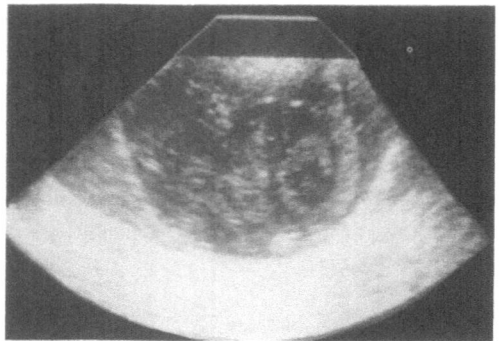

Fig. 6.9. 43-year-old woman examined for hepatosplenomegaly: several hydatid lesions were found in the liver. Note the type IV appearance of the splenic hydatid cyst

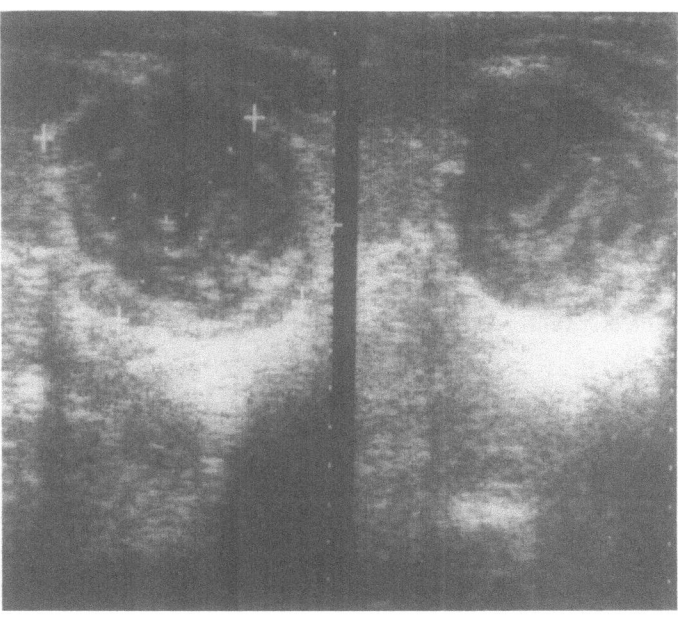

Fig. 6.10. Hydatid cyst in a 44-year-old man: type IV. The membranes folded inside the cyst create a ribbon appearance

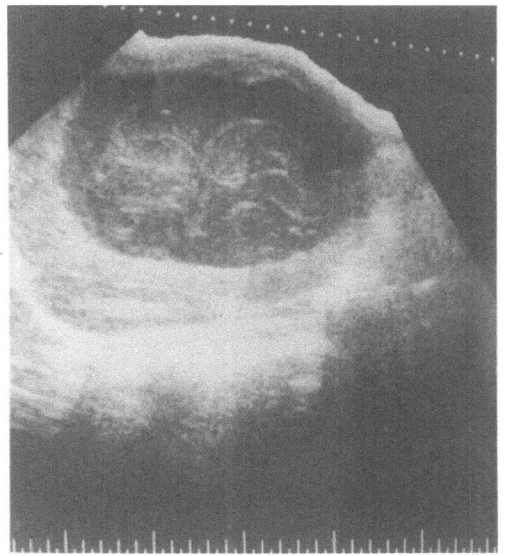

Fig. 6.11. Hydatid cyst in a 40-year-old woman: type IV. Note the ribbon-like appearance of the membranes folded inside the cyst

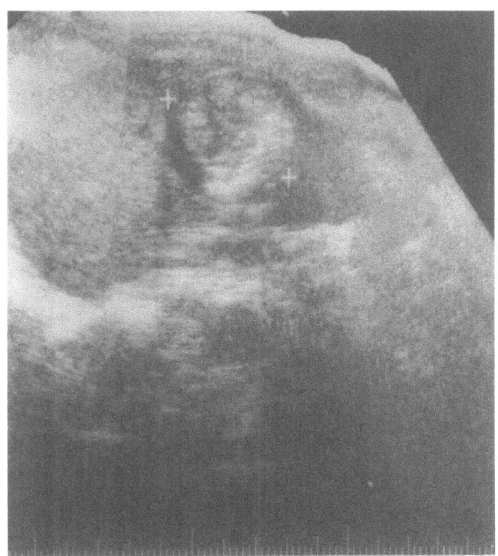

Fig. 6.12. 63-year-old woman with a solid, 5 cm diameter hydatid cyst with partial wall calcification: type IV

They correspond to reorganized, occasionally infected, cysts. Determination of the etiology of such lesions is difficult: sonographic data is almost never sufficient and there are numerous differential diagnoses.

Type V: Cysts with Thick, Reflective Walls (Figs. 6.14 and 6.15). Defects with a hyperechoic, convex contour, and a posterior acoustic shadow (produced by echo reflection off the cyst wall) represent calcified hydatid cysts.

Such patterns are rarely observed in children. The diagnosis can easily be confirmed by a plain abdominal film.

Along with its capacity to identify the various patterns of hydatid cysts, ultrasonography has several other indications:

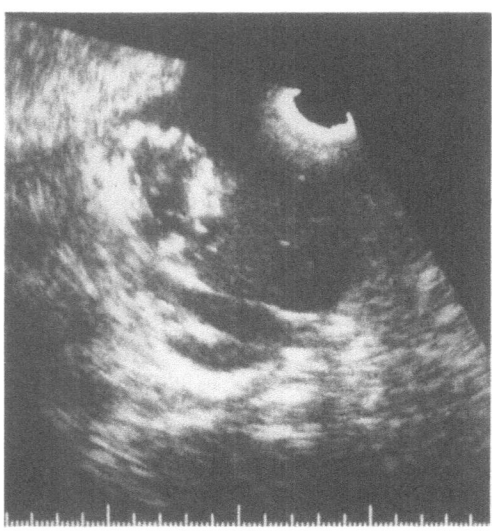

Fig. 6.15. Calcified hydatid cyst: type V

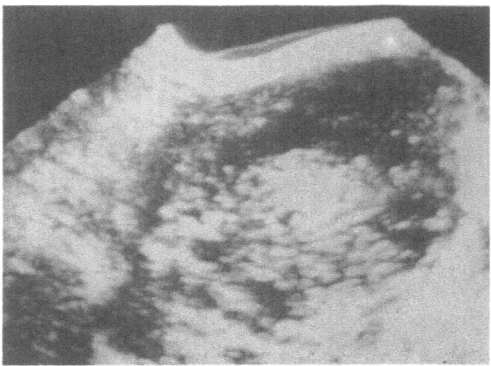

Fig. 6.13. Hydatid cyst in a 60-year old woman visualized as a large inhomogeneous mass: type IV

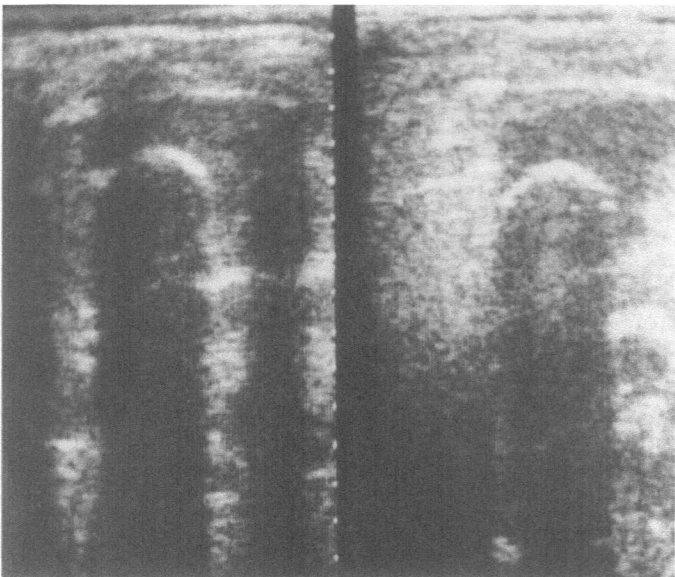

Fig. 6.14. Calcified hydatid cyst: type V

- Diagnosis of postoperative complications (essentially infection)
- Evaluation of compression of contiguous structures by an enlarging cyst (upper pole of the left kidney, left hemidiaphragm, aorta, left liver, etc.)
- Assessment of possible cystic rupture, particularly into the lungs through the left hemidiaphragm (rare)

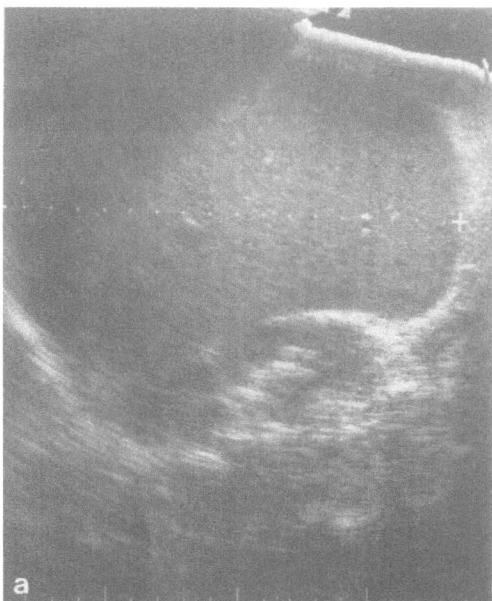

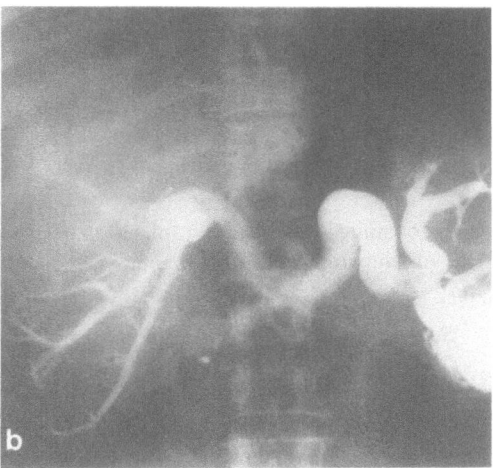

Fig. 6.16a, b. Hepatic hydatid cyst compressing the left portal branch causing portal hypertension with homogeneous splenomegaly. Splenic sonogram (**a**) and splenoportograph (**b**)

- Investigation of portal hypertension secondary to portal system compression by hepatic hydatid lesions (Fig. 6.16)

Intrasplenic hydatid cysts are often easily located, but once they reach a certain size (over 10 cm) it may prove difficult to determine whether they arise in the spleen, the upper pole of the left kidney, or the left lobe of the liver. However, topographic imprecisions of the sort have little or no consequence on patient management.

6.1.1.2 Alveolar Hydatid Disease

General Features. Much rarer than unilocular hydatidosis, alveolar disease is caused by *Echinococcus multilocularis*. The adult resides in the intestine of foxes and dogs, the definitive hosts. In man, the larvae are responsible for severe lesions owing to their noncystic nature. The liver is the main site of predilection, followed by the lungs. The prognosis is generally poor. Alveolar hydatid disease is limited to cold and mountainous regions of the northern hemisphere (Alaska, Canada, Siberia, southern Germany, Switzerland).

Man is infected by consuming wild berries that have been contaminated by the excreta of infected foxes or other wild canidae, or by handling the carcasses of such animals (hunters, forest wardens, animal raisers). The spleen is rarely affected, and those cases that do occur probably result from arterial hematogenous dissemination.

Sonographic Features. The larval stage of *E. multilocularis* differs considerably from the hydatid; the sonographic pattern of alveolar hydatid disease is thus quite different from that of hydatidosis. Because the growth pattern of unilocular cysts resembles that of malignant tumors, there are a number of differential diagnoses (Weill 1980). Owing to the infrequency of splenic alveolar hydatids, diagnosis by ultrasound alone is nearly impossible.

6.1.2 Histoplasmosis

6.1.2.1 General Features

When disseminated along hematogenous or lymphatic pathways, mycoses often result in multiorgan lesions, with the spleen being a favored site. Lesions generally manifest as a mycotic splenic abscess or fairly homogeneous splenomegaly (Chulay and Lankeran 1976; Dubbins 1980; Miller et al. 1982; Page et al. 1980). Histoplasmosis is the most frequent of those mycoses that invariably involve the spleen, and it occurs in numerous regions of the world (North and South America, the Middle East, Central and South Africa, the Pacific). Two forms of this fungus have been identified: American histoplasmosis, caused by *Histoplasma capsulatum,* and African histoplasmosis, due to *H. duboisii.* Only *H. capsulatum* has a particular affinity for the reticuloendothelial system. The lungs are the most frequent site of involvement.

Clinical Manifestations. The primary infection is usually asymptomatic, and generally occurs in the lungs. Mild pulmonary symptoms are frequent after an incubation period of 7 to 21 days. Spontaneous clinical and radiologic healing is the rule after several weeks. Spotty microcalcifications in the lungs and occasionally the spleen permit retrospective diagnosis. In rare instances, severe disease develops when the parasite spreads by hematogenous or lymphatic seeding to the entire reticuloendothelial system. Acute disseminated histoplasmosis results in multiorgan lesions (including splenic sites) and fever, and is usually lethal without treatment.

6.1.2.2 Sonographic Features

Ultrasonography may demonstrate homogeneous splenomegaly. On occasion, the classic microcalcifications of histoplasmosis (Dubuisson and Jones 1983) will be visualized as echodense defects with posterior shadowing.

6.1.3 Amebiasis

6.1.3.1 General Features

The protozoa responsible for amebiasis are widely distributed throughout the world, affecting around 10% of the population, generally asymptomatically. Of the many amebas that parasite man, only *Entamoeba histolytica* (hematophagus ameba) is pathogenic. Commonly found in the colon, where it causes amebic dysentery, *E. histolytica* can spread to the liver and thence to the lungs, the usual site of complications in amebiases. Splenic involvement is exceptional, occurring by hematogenous dissemination of the parasite or direct extension from the left colic flexure.

6.1.3.2 Sonographic Features

Although the sonographic appearance of splenic amebiasis has not yet been described, it should probably correspond to those of hepatic amebic abscesses: semisolid defects in the nonsuppurative phase and fluid collections after liquefaction necrosis. Several other unusual hepatic images have also been reported (De Dios-Vega et al. 1977; Pawar et al. 1982; Peyron et al. 1981). The rarity of splenic amebiasis makes ultrasound diagnosis difficult; clinical and biological examinations are required.

6.2 Splenic Lesions Secondary to Hepatic Parasitoses

6.2.1 Schistosomiasis

Schistosomiasis is a helminthiasis caused by one of four trematodes of the genus *Schistosoma:*

- *S. haematobium,* found mainly in Africa (Egypt, Madagascar) and southwest Asia; the intermediate host is a snail
- *S. mansoni,* occurring primarily in tropical South America (Venezuela, Brazil) and Africa, while several small areas of occurrence have been reported in southern Portugal and Spain; the intermediate host is a snail
- *S. japonicum,* generally confined to Chile,

Japan, Korea, and the Philippines; the intermediate host is an amphibious fresh water snail
- *S. intercalatum,* which is found only in Africa; the intermediate host is a snail

6.2.1.1 General Features

Man is infected when fork-tailed cercaria escape from the intermediate host into water and penetrate the skin. Carried into the general circulation, the young schistosomes dwell exclusively in the mesenteric and pelvic venules. After approximately 1 week, surviving schistosomes establish themselves in the portal system; they reach maturity in the venous branches after some 20 days. The first eggs are produced after approximately 60 days. Certain eggs remain in the surrounding tissues where they cause a granulomatous tissue reaction; others are carried in the bloodstream throughout the entire body (Kane and Katz 1982; Lapierre 1974; Laverdant et al. 1980; Leger et al. 1973; Phillips et al. 1975).

S. mansoni and *S. japonicum* are responsible for most splenic lesions. Prominent features include:

- Formation of splenic granulomas resembling clusters of vesicles varying from 1 to several millimeters in size; lesions of this type have been reported in 18.7% of patients with digestive tract schistosomiasis explored by laparoscopy (Laverdant 1982).
- Splenomegaly secondary to the portal hypertension that occurs in this parasitosis (the granulomata cause fibrosis in the portal spaces leading to presinusoidal occlusion). This fibrosis is never accompanied by regenerative nodules (Aubry et al. 1980). Portal hypertension gradually increases in severity, causing splenomegaly, prehepatic venous stasis, etc.

S. haematobium essentially affects the genitourinary tract. Hepatic lesions are rare, although the parasite can cause the extensive chronic splenic enlargement encountered in endemic regions ("Egyptian" splenomegaly).

S. intercalatum basically affects the rectum; hepatosplenic involvement is rarely reported.

The clinical manifestations of schistosomiasis depend on the type of parasite and the stage of the disease:

- The initial phase of contamination is signalled by transient and very mild cutaneous irritations that may go unnoticed.
- The toxemic phase is characterized by reactions of an immune-allergic nature: fever, hepatosplenomegaly, "asthmatic" dyspnea, neurologic disorders.
- The intestinal phase, corresponding to the release of eggs, occurs after approximately 3 months. Depending on the parasite, clinical manifestations are urinary or intestinal in nature. Portal hypertension, the most dangerous complication of digestive tract schistosomiasis, develops more or less rapidly after episodes of diarrhea and deterioration in general condition (hepatosplenic phase).

6.2.1.2 Sonographic Features
     (Figs. 6.17 and 6.18)

Individuals with splenic involvement by schistosomiasis usually have more or less homogeneous splenomegaly, but the actual degree of organ enlargement varies. The spleen often retains smooth contours, but nodular defects have been reported as well (7% of cases for Cerri et al. 1984). The small granulations ob-

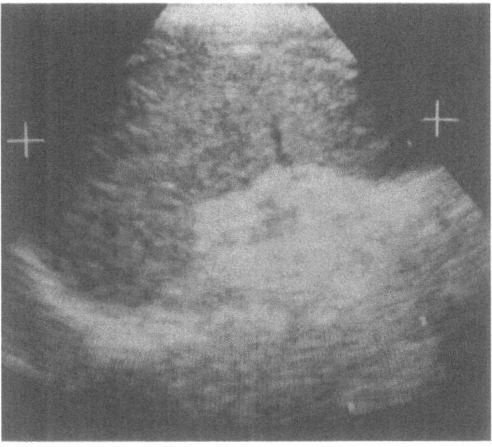

Fig. 6.17. Large homogeneous splenomegaly in a patient with hepatic schistosomiasis

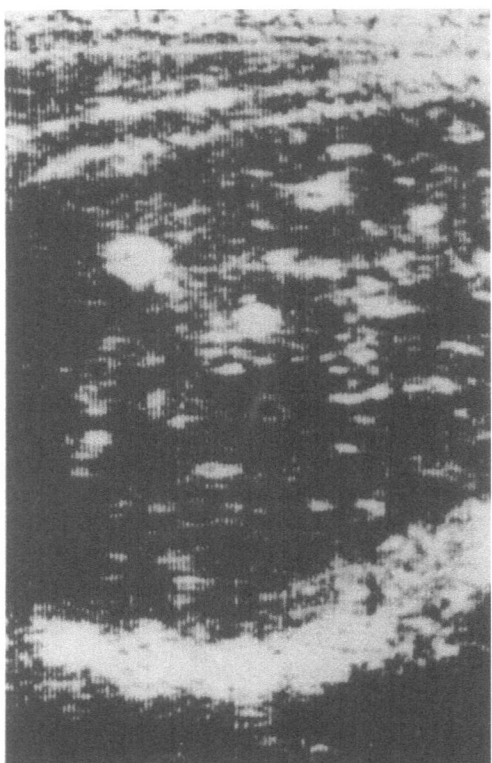

Fig. 6.18. Multiple echogenic nodules of schistosomiasis in an enlarged spleen. (Courtesy of Dr. Cerri)

served at laparoscopy have no sonographic equivalent. The splenic vein, the splenomesenteric axis, and the portal vein show varying degrees of enlargement, a consequence of portal hypertension. The high incidence of associated left hepatic lobe enlargement and right lobe atrophy facilitates investigation (Cerri et al. 1984). Sonography can also demonstrate the other signs of portal hypertension (hepatofibrosis, ascites, etc.).

Doppler ultrasonography permits the diagnosis of portal hypertension; this technique also allows evaluation of splenic volume and the status of the portal vein–splenic vein axis after medical treatment or surgery (diameter and permeability of spontaneous or surgically created anastomoses). Splenic cysts can also be detected during such investigations (Capdeville et al. 1978).

6.3 Nonspecific Homogeneous Splenomegaly

This section covers the main etiologies of nonspecific splenic lesions occurring in parasitoses. Ultrasound features include varying degrees of splenomegaly, usually with a homogeneous echo pattern. Sonolucent patterns are occasionally observed; chronically enlarged spleens may demonstrate increased echogenicity. The contours of the spleen are smooth. No specific appearances have been reported. Ultrasonography can be performed to search for those rare instances of associated portal hypertension.

6.3.1 Malaria

6.3.1.1 General Features

Malaria, a disease of red blood cells, is caused by a protozoan of the genus *Plasmodium*. Transmitted by the bite of female mosquitoes of the genus *Anopheles*, malaria remains a serious disease in many parts of the world, especially in the tropics and subtropics (Latin America, South America, the Sahara, Asia; Wyler 1983). It has been estimated that over 1 billion persons are affected worldwide, and malaria-related deaths are put at over 1 million annually.

Malaria produces several different clinical pictures:

- Primary attacks: after a period of incubation lasting 5–20 days, continuous fever develops, accompanied by nausea, vomiting, and often intense headache. Hepatomegaly may occur, but the spleen remains normal. Splenomegaly is a late manifestation of spontaneous termination, and thus a favorable prognostic factor in nontreated patients.
- Periodic paroxysms: The clinical pictures of tertian and quartan malaria have been extensively described and allow easy diagnosis. Splenomegaly is common.
- Pernicious syndromes may occur at any age, but most patients are children aged 4 months to 4 years. Cerebral malaria, characterized by acute encephalopathy, is usually lethal. Moderate splenomegaly of late on-

set occurs in one-third of cases: it reflects a defensive reaction of the body's reticuloendothelial system and as such is associated with a favorable outcome.
- Chronic malaria occurs in individuals continually exposed to repeated infection without chemoprophylaxis. The disease associates anemia with asthenia, edema, splenomegaly, and a low fever (around 38 °C), and responds well to medical treatment.

As splenomegaly is a nearly constant feature in malaria, it can be used as the basis for evaluation of the degree of infestation in endemic zones. The splenic index is defined as the number of cases of splenomegaly per 100 individuals examined: hypoendemic area 0–10 cases; mesoendemic area 11–50; hyperendemic area 51–75; and holoendemic area >76.

6.3.1.2 Sonographic Features

Ultrasonography is of limited interest for malaria as the disease is diagnosed clinically and biologically. When doubt persists, ultrasound can confirm the homogeneous, solitary nature of splenomegaly.

6.3.2 Leishmaniasis (Kala Azar)

6.3.2.1 General Features

Leishmaniases are zoonotic infections caused by flagellated protozoa of the genus *Leishmania*. Transmitted by the bite of a hematophagous insect (the female sandfly), these endocellular parasites attack the reticuloendothelial system of vertebrate hosts. While three different species infect man, only *L. donovani* causes visceral leishmaniasis, or kala azar, with splenic involvement. The other two species cause cutaneous and mucocutaneous lesions.

The intermediate vector, a sandfly varying in length from 2–3 mm, thrives in warm regions. It is active all year long in intertropical areas and during the warm season in temperate zones. Kala azar occurs in several regions of the world: central Africa, along the Mediterranean, Middle East, southwest Asia, and South America. Disease in children is usually differentiated from the adult form.

Infantile kala azar, the most frequent form in the Mediterranean region, affects children under age 4. After a generally insidious period of incubation, the clinical picture reflects gradual deterioration in general status accompanied by constant fever with a hectic course. Enormous, nontender smooth and mobile splenomegaly reaching or extending beyond the umbilicus is common. The liver is enlarged but nontender, without ascites or jaundice. Deep adenopathies may be present. The disease is usually fatal unless treated.

Adult visceral leishmaniasis, occurring in India, China, South America, and subsaharan Africa, resembles childhood disease except that hepatosplenic involvement is less marked. Deterioration of the general condition is accompanied by cutaneous signs (hyperpigmentation), digestive disorders, and a hemorrhagic syndrome. The course is fatal without therapy.

6.3.2.2 Sonographic Features

Ultrasonography is of little value once the diagnosis has been made. It can confirm the existence of splenomegaly and homogeneous hepatomegaly, but there are no specific patterns (Fig. 6.19).

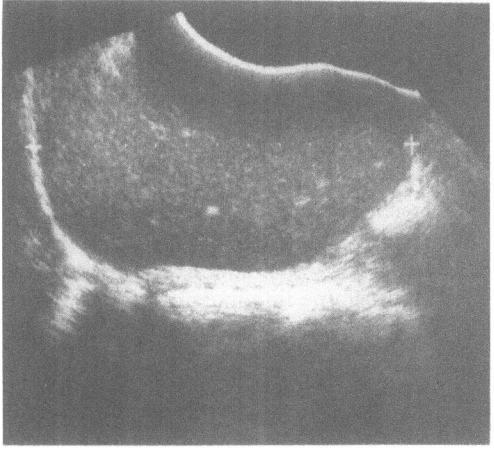

Fig. 6.19. Splenomegaly during infantile kala azar

6.3.3 Toxoplasmosis

This cosmopolitan anthrozoonotic infection is caused by *Toxoplasma gondii (Eimeriidean sporozoairean),* an intracellular protozoan with an elective trophism for the reticuloendothelial system (Ben Rachid and Blaha 1970; Manigand et al. 1975). Human toxoplasmosis occurs in two distinct forms: congenital infection transmitted through the placenta, and acquired infection, seen in both children and adults.

6.3.3.1 Congenital Toxoplasmosis

Although the disease remains latent in the majority of cases, clinical manifestations vary with the severity of infestation and the date of infection during pregnancy. Infections occurring in the first trimester cause the most severe and generalized lesions. The infected neonate may present with either disseminated infection or acute nervous system involvement. Splenic involvement occurs in both disseminated disease and mild infections, and is accompanied by jaundice, hepatomegaly, convulsions, and a hemorrhagic syndrome. Disseminated disease has a poor prognosis.

Ultrasonography is of little use for this parasitosis, aside from confirming homogeneous splenomegaly. Literature reports mention histologic detection of numerous necrotic foci and rare parasitic groups in endothelial cells, but there is no sonographic equivalent.

6.3.3.2 Acquired Toxoplasmosis

Infection generally goes unnoticed and is detected only by blood tests. Severe forms are rare, although rapidly fatal multiorgan involvement can occur in immunocompromised individuals and patients with neoplastic disease. Splenic sonograms cannot demonstrate the innumerable inflammatory foci, reflecting local reactions, or the presence of parasite cells.

6.3.4 Trypanosomiasis

6.3.4.1 General Features

Human trypanosomiasis is caused by a hemoflagellate of the genus *Trypanosoma.* Two distinct types of human trypanosomes have been identified on the basis of their clinical manifestations and geographic distribution: American trypanosomes, which cause Chagas' disease, and African trypanosomes, seen essentially in subsaharan Africa, responsible for sleeping sickness. Splenic involvement occurs only with the African form, and is both frequent and massive.

After an incubation period of 10-20 days, during which symptoms may be very mild or even go unnoticed, the disease enters a febrile phase. In the initial period of parasite dissemination to the lymphatic system and the bloodstream, the trypanosomes affect the entire reticuloendothelial system. Physical findings include hepatomegaly, adenopathies, cutaneous manifestations, and fever. Moderate splenomegaly occurs early in the disease course. In the absence of treatment, the disease enters a terminal stage: the parasites attack the central nervous system (cerebral trypanosomiasis), causing the characteristic sleeping sickness syndrome.

6.3.4.2 Sonographic Features

Ultrasound is of little utility for diagnosis, but will demonstrate the homogeneous nature of any splenic enlargement.

6.3.5 Idiopathic Splenomegaly

Idiopathic (Mediterranean or tropical) splenomegaly is a clinical and biological entity defined by a constellation of more or less specific criteria:

- Splenomegaly with no recognized etiology
- Hypersplenism and histologic modification of the spleen
- Liver involvement, varying from a normal liver to confirmed cirrhosis
- Biological disorders (coagulopathy, generally elevated immunoglobulin level)

This type of splenomegaly has been reported in tropical regions, the Mediterranean area, and around Los Angeles. The exact etiology of such splenic enlargement remains unclear, but a parasitic origin is probable. When cirrhosis develops, the spleen may present the signs of Banti's syndrome, a currently controversial entity.

Approximately 75% of all cases of chronic splenomegaly in tropical regions have no recognized etiology, but the incidence is declining as progress is made in diagnostic procedures. Infectious disease (tuberculosis), parasitic disease (mycoses, malaria, leishmaniasis, etc.), viral infections, hematologic disorders, and toxic phenomena are increasingly cited as the probable cause. The sensitivity of such nonspecific splenomegaly to antimalarial drugs and the presence of specific plasmatic immunologic signs has led certain authors to suggest a malarial origin. Ultrasonographic examination of the spleen of such patients is extremely helpful as the technique can determine the homogeneous nature of enlargement and evaluate any associated signs, and in particular portal hypertension (Fig. 6.20).

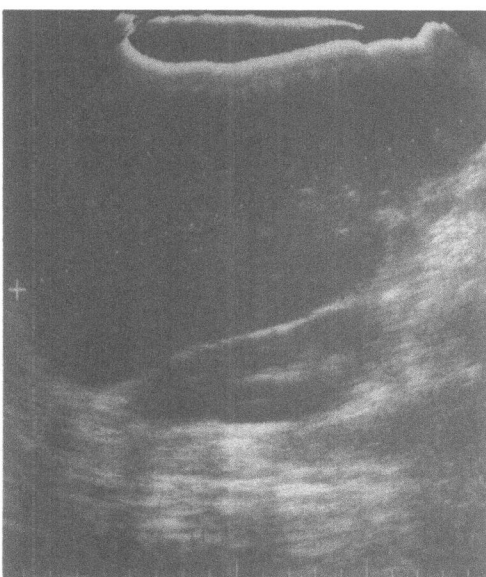

Fig. 6.20. Chronic homogeneous splenomegaly of undetermined origin

6.4 Conclusion

Splenic involvement in parasitoses manifests most often as splenomegaly. However, even in those regions where parasitic diseases are endemic, there are many other possible causes for splenomegaly: infectious diseases, hematologic disorders, portal hypertension, trauma, obesity, etc. (Table 6.1). The indications for splenic ultrasonography vary widely: the technique is primordial for investigation of hydatid pathologies because the sonographic patterns can suggest the diagnosis; it is less helpful for the investigation of chronic splenomegaly (Gharbi et al. 1985; Pascal-Suisse et al. 1980; Shirkhoda et al. 1980).

Used in combination with clinical and biological examinations, splenic ultrasonography can:

- Affirm the existence of splenomegaly, evaluate the extent of involvement, and make the differential diagnosis by ruling out other left upper quadrant masses (affecting the liver or kidney, for example)
- Suggest the etiology for hydatid cysts, and occasionally for amebiasis, schistosomiasis, and trypanosomiasis with portal hypertension (Tables 6.2 and 6.3)
- Guide puncture biopsy when accurate diagnosis is desirable (Solbiati et al. 1983)
- Detect associated involvement in other abdominal organs (Laurin and Kaude 1984)
- Evaluate response to treatment and detect possible iatrogenic complications

Table 6.1. Major causes of parasitic splenomegaly

Acute febrile splenomegaly	Malaria Kala azar Schistosomiasis Histoplasmosis Toxoplasmosis Trypanosomiasis
Chronic splenomegaly	Idiopathic splenomegaly (Mediterranean and tropical) Schistosomiasis Hydatid cyst

Table 6.2. Value of ultrasonography for the investigation of parasitic spleens

Parasitosis	Frequency of splenic involvement	Sonographic features	Specificity of ultrasound	Value of ultrasound
Echinococcus granulosus	+	Type I–IV (hydatid cyst)	+ + +	+ + +
Echinococcus multilocularis	Rare	Pseudotumoral	+ +	+ + +
Amebiasis	Rare	Abscess	+ +	+ + +
Malaria	+ + +	Homogeneous splenomegaly	+	+
Leishmaniasis	+ + +	Homogeneous splenomegaly	+	+
Toxoplasmosis	+ +	Homogeneous splenomegaly	+	+
Trypanosomiasis	+ + +	Homogeneous splenomegaly	+	+
Schistosomiasis	+ + +	Homogeneous splenomegaly +, portal hypertension +, nodules	+ +	+ + +
Histoplasmosis	+ + +	Homogeneous splenomegaly	+	+

Table 6.3. Ultrasound diagnosis of splenic involvement

Sonographic pattern	Fluid collection	Separated membrane	Septated fluid collection	Portal hypertension	Homogeneous splenomegaly	Inhomogeneous splenomegaly ± calcifications
Parasitic etiology	Hydatid cyst (Type I)	Hydatid cyst (Type II)	Hydatid cyst (Type III)	Schistosomiasis Hydatid cyst	Malaria Leishmaniasis Toxoplasmosis Trypanosomiasis Histoplasmosis Mediterranean or tropical	Hydatid cyst (IV, V) Alveolar hydatid disease Schistosomiasis Amebiasis Histoplasmosis
Other etiologies	Epidermoid cyst Pseudocystic hematoma		Cystic lymphangioma	Cirrhosis Vascular obstruction	Hemopathy Infection Tumor Other	Hematoma Tumor Infarction Other

When combined with the immunologic tests that have become routine practice, ultrasound examination of the spleen can shorten the interval preceding diagnosis in difficult cases; the technique thus has great potential for development in areas of endemic parasitoses.

6.5 References

Aubry P, Capdeville P, Durand G (1980) Les manifestations hépato-spléniques des bilharzioses. Médecine Tropicale 40: 53–57

Ben Rachid MS, Blaha R (1970) La toxoplasmose humaine et animale en Tunisie. Tunisie Médicale 48: 101–110

Capdeville P, Legars A, Delprat J, Pons R (1978) Kyste de la rate chez un bilharzien: découverte par laparoscopie. Médecine Tropicale 38: 81–84

Cerri GG, Alves VAF, Magalhães A (1984) Hepatosplenic schistosomiasis mansoni: ultrasound manifestations. Radiology 153: 777–780

Chulay JD, Lankerani MR (1976) Splenic abscess. 61: 513-522

De Dios-Vega JF, Muro J, Pérez-Jimenez F, Segura JM, Ortiz-Vazquez J (1977) Valor de los ultrasonidos en el diagnostico de los quistes histadicos hepaticos. Estudio de 31 casos. Rev Clin Esp 144: 37-42

Dubbins PA (1980) Ultrasound in the diagnosis of splenic abscess. Br J Radiol 53: 488-489

Dubuisson RL, Jones TB (1983) Splenic abscess due to blastomycosis: scintigraphic, sonographic and CT evaluation. AJR 140: 66-68

Dupuy JP, Catanzano G, Bouchet JB (1984) Le lymphangiome kystique hépato-splénique. Ann Radiol 27: 417-420

Gharbi HA, Hassine W, Brauner MW, Dupuch K (1981) Ultrasound examination of the hydatic liver. Radiology 139: 459-463

Gharbi HA, Hassine W, Abdesselem K (1985) L'hydatidose abdominale à l'échographie: réflexions et aspects particuliers (Echinococcus granulosus). Ann Radiol 28: 31-34

Hassine W, Dupuch K, Gharbi HA (1980) Apport de l'échotomographie dans la pathologie hydatique du foie chez l'enfant. J Radiol 61: 323-327

Horchani A, Hassine W, Gharbi HA, Saied H, Ayed M, Zmerli S (1983) Apport de l'échotomographie dans le diagnostic du kyste hydatique du rein: à propos de 43 cas vérifiés. J Urol Nephrol 89: 515-520

Karle RA, Katz SG (1982) The spectrum of sonographic findings in portal hypertension: a subject review and new observations. Radiology 142: 453-458

King DL (1973) Ultrasonography of echinococcal cysts. J Clin Ultrasound 1: 64-67

Lapierre J (1974) Bilharziose hépatosplénique. Pathogénie générale. Diagnostic biologique. Indications thérapeutiques. Ann Gastroentérol Hépatol 10: 341-353

Laurin S, Kaude JV (1984) Diagnosis of liver-spleen abscesses in children with emphasis on ultrasound for the initial and follow-up examination. Pediatr Radiol 14: 198-204

Laverdant C (1982) Aspects diagnostiques et évolutifs des bilharzioses digestives à leur phase d'invasion. Bull Acad Nat Méd 166: 627-632

Laverdant C, Thabaut A, Hardelin J, Cristau P, Molinie C, Durosoir JL, Essioux H, Daly JP, Larroque P, Cathalan G (1980) Les bilharzioses africaines de première invasion: éléments de diagnostic, évolution à 5 ans. Médecine Tropicale 40: 251-258

Leger L, Sors C, Benhammou JP, Boutelier T, Hernandez C, Le Aigre G (1973) Bilharziose hépatosplénique et hypertension portale. Presse Med 25: 1275-1278

Lewall DB, McCorkell SJ (1985) Hepatic echinococcal cysts: Sonographic appearance and classification. Radiology 155: 773-775

Manigand G, Couzineau P, Foulon D, Bodak A, Deparis M (1975) Toxoplasmose acquise aigüe fébrile de l'adulte sain à forme typhoïde. Sem Hôp Paris 51: 1181-1184

Matossian RM, Rickard MD, Smyth JD (1977) Hydatidosis: a global problem of increasing importance. Bull OMS 55: 499-507

Miller JH, Greenfield LD, Wald BR (1982) Candidiasis of the liver and spleen in childhood. Radiology 142: 375-380

Page CP, Coltman CA, Robertson HD, Nelson EA (1980) Candidal abscess of the spleen in patients with acute leukemia. Surg Gyn Obstet 151: 604-608

Pascal-Suisse P, Marbot P, Peyron JP (1980) L'échographie: principes, techniques and application à la pathologie tropicale et parasitaire. Médecine Tropicale 40: 197-210

Pawar S, Kay CJ, Gonzalez R, Taylor KJW, Rosenfield AT (1982) Sonography of splenic abscess. AJR 138: 259-262

Peyron JP, Pascal-Suisse P, Marbot P (1981) Abcès amibien du foie: aspects échographiques inhabituels. JEMU 2: 235-238

Phillips JF, Cockrill H, Jorge E, Steiner R (1975) Radiographic evaluation of patients with schistosomiasis. Radiology 114: 31-37

Rao BK, AuBuchon J, Lieberman LM, Polcyn RE (1981) Cystic lymphangiomatosis of the spleen: a radio-pathologic correlation. Radiology 141: 781-782

Shirkhoda A, McCartney WH, Staab EV, Mittelstaedt CA (1980) Imaging of the spleen: a proposed algorithm. AJR 135: 195-198

Solbiati L, Bossi MC, Bellotti E, Ravetto C, Montali G (1983) Focal lesions in the spleen: sonographic patterns and guided biopsy. AJR 140: 53-69

Weill FS (1980) L'ultrasonographie en pathologie digestive. Vigot, Paris

Wyler DJ (1983) Splenic functions in malaria. Lymphology 16: 121-127

7 Subject Index

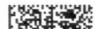